W9-ACC-312

Light Style

Light Style

The New American Cuisine

The Low Calorie, Low Salt, Low Fat Way to Good Food and Good Health

Rose Dosti, Deborah Kidushim, & Mark Wolke

Illustrations by Heather Preston
Photographs by Hans Albers

1817

Harper & Row, Publishers, San Francisco
Cambridge, Hagerstown, New York, Philadelphia
London, Mexico City, São Paulo, Sydney

A portion of this book originally appeared in *Bon Appetit* magazine.

Light Style: The New American Cuisine. Copyright ©1979 by Rose Dosti, Deborah Kidushim, Mark Wolke. All rights reserved. Printed in the United States of America. No part of this book may be used or reproduced in any manner whatsoever without written permission except in the case of brief quotations embodied in critical articles and reviews. For information address Harper & Row, Publishers, Inc., 10 East 53rd Street, New York, NY 10022. Published simultaneously in Canada by Fitzhenry & Whiteside, Limited, Toronto.

First Harper & Row paperback edition published 1982

Designed by Patricia Girvin Dunbar

Library of Congress Cataloging in Publication Data

Dosti, Rose.
    Light style, the new American cuisine.

    Bibliography: p. 305
    Includes index.
    1. Cookery, American.   2. Sugar-free diet — Recipes.   3. Salt-free diet —
Recipes.   4. Low-fat diet — Recipes.   I. Kidushim, Deborah, joint author.
II. Wolke, Mark, joint author.   III. Title.
TX715.D6875   1979   641.5'63   79-1771
ISBN 0-06-250487-8

86 10 9 8 7 6 5 4

Contents

Acknowledgments

We are grateful to all the people who helped in the preparation of this book. In particular, we would like to acknowledge the generous help of Mo Ezzani, Josie Wilson, Ramona Ponce and Edwin Smith, who worked in the testing and development of the recipes. We also thank Kathy DeKarr and Marya Dosti for testing many of the recipes.

Special thanks to Professor Roslyn B. Alfin-Slater, Ph.D., chairman of the Department of Nutritional Sciences at UCLA, for reviewing our manuscript and for her invaluable comments.

For their support, we thank Ralph S. Saul, chairman, Insurance Company of North America, Philip Shapiro, vice-president, and Saul Goldfarb, regional director, Hospital Affiliates, International, Inc., Arthur Michelson, administrator of Queen of Angels Hospital in Los Angeles, and Gershon Lesser, M.D., J.D.

Our appreciation goes to Hans Albers for creating the beautiful photographs in the book.

Introduction:
The New American Cuisine

Light Style is a new concept of cooking and eating. It is the New American Cuisine of low calories, low fat, low cholesterol, low salt, and low sugar. And it's for practically everyone.

It's the cuisine of preventive health and nutrition awareness for those who want to stay healthy. It's also the scientific cuisine of dietary change for those who need to modify their diet for medical reasons.

Light Style is the American cuisine of simplicity, glamor, and good taste. The recipes, in fact, are so delicious you won't believe the calories are so low and nutritional value so high.

We wrote *Light Style* because, as observers and participants in the health world, we have been made deeply aware that people need to be shown *how* to lower calories, fat, cholesterol, and salt in their daily cooking. One of the biggest dietary problems in America is not the acceptance of dietary change, but how to do it!

For decades, the health community has been pointing out that Americans eat too much fat, salt, and sugar, and consume too many calories. Scientists have recommended changes in the American diet that they believe may help prevent heart disease, cancer, stroke, obesity, and diabetes. But little has been done on a mass scale to *teach* people *how* to revise eating habits. The scientific community talks about change without providing the formula. It's like having the menu with no recipes. No interpretation. Nothing to show Americans how to change everyday eating habits.

The RDA (Recommended Dietary Allowances) provided by the National Academy of Sciences as a standard for good nutrition has been available for many years, but it is too difficult for the layman to decipher. The Basic Four Food Group concept that grew out of the RDA as a guide for implementing the standards is also difficult to apply without guidance.

Even the more recent U.S. Senate Select Committee on Dietary Goals, which presented the American people with recommendations for dietary reform, offered little interpretive help. The Goals were based on recommendations of some scientists to decrease nutrients that in some cases were thought to be related to chronic diseases in this country. It was suggested that Americans avoid becoming overweight by consuming only as many calories as they expended, increasing intake of complex carbohydrates and naturally-occurring sugar derived from fruits, vegetables, and grains, and decreasing processed sugars in the diet. The Committee recommended that Americans reduce their overall fat intake, consuming equal amounts of saturated, monounsaturated, and polyunsaturated fats. A reduction of cholesterol intake (except for children, young women, and older adults), as well as reductions in sodium and protein, also were recommended.

But the recommendations did not show *how* to apply such reforms in daily cooking and eating habits.

Light Style does. *Light Style* shows *scientifically* how the New American Cuisine of low calories, fat, cholesterol, salt, and sugar actually works. It attempts to show *why* the New American Cuisine is the cuisine of preventive health and nutrition awareness by providing not only recipes, but also nutritional information that we believe to be a necessary tool for dietary reform. We have tried to stress simplicity and beauty and create recipes that are delicious and nutritious, yet low in calories, fats, cholesterol, and salt.

And *Light Style* is for practically everyone. It's for those who want to use it as a preventative health measure as well as those whose dietary restrictions demand strict change. It can create the necessary awareness for making proper food choices and put the dieter in the driver's seat at last.

The key to the New American Cuisine as presented in *Light Style* is recipe modification, so that anyone can adjust and adapt their recipes to conform to his or her individual need. The chapter on Modifying Recipes (p. 253) provides the tools for making necessary ingredient changes, whether you wish to increase or decrease calories, fats, sugar, cholesterol, or salt. We urge you to make good use of the information.

The recipes themselves contain a nutrient analysis of calories, sodium, fat, cholesterol, and so-called "Diabetic Exchange" for diabetics who must carefully calculate simple carbohydrate calories in their diets. The diabetic exchange analysis in each recipe is based on the traditional exchange list as a convenience to those who are still working with it. Those who wish to use the exchange list recently developed by the American Diabetic Association may easily convert the information by referring to their own list.

The recipes also offer options for either increasing or decreasing values of these nutrients. Numerous tables and charts are available for most any type of recipe modification.

How do *Light Style* recipes cut calories, sodium, fat, and cholesterol?

Calories

We hope that *Light Style* will teach the reader to think of calories in terms of the nutrients they provide and not simply as calories. It's the total nutrient intake and not the total calories that count.

There are several ways *Light Style* cuts calories. *Light Style* recipes teach portion control, one of the key elements of calorie control. Recommended portions in the recipes are based on the USDA suggestions for serving sizes in all Basic Four Food Groups (milk group, meat group, bread group, and fruit-vegetable group). People of different ages, however, have different caloric requirements. Children, the elderly, and pregnant women require more nutrient-dense calories to compensate for their special needs. One complaint about the Committee on Dietary Goals is that they failed to detail the special dietary needs for these groups.

Children who need extra calories for their growing bodies and high energy expenditure should be assured of a healthy array of foods rich in both nutrients and calories. Whole milk instead of nonfat milk, and even occasional sweets, can provide the extra calories children need. Less active and overweight children should be encouraged to eat less of the simple carbohydrates and add some form of exercise to their daily routines. For these children, *Light Style* becomes an effective calorie-lowering, nutrient-dense tool for weight reduction. *Light Style* is also a blessing for the elderly, whose nutrient needs increase while calorie needs diminish.

Our recipes make use of so-called "low-calorie margarine" which is actually margarine whipped with water to create double its volume. Because you are actually using less margarine (about half when used in equivalent amounts) you are consuming half the calories. You may use the commercially whipped margarine, referred to as "low-calorie" margarine on the package label, or our home recipe which not only saves money but also is free of preservatives and salt, if you start out with the unsalted product. A recipe for whipped butter, which also reduces the calories of butter by half when used in equivalent amounts, is also given.

We offer as options some specialty products in our recipes that make cutting calories easier. For example, fructose, a natural fruit sugar available in crystalline or liquid form, is given for its calorie-lowering effect. It is one-and-one-half times sweeter than sugar, which means that less is needed for sweetening. Calories, therefore, drop by at least half when using fructose in place of sugar. Fructose also helps enhance and compensate for flavors missing in unsalted foods.

Although artificial sweeteners are not encouraged because of their proclaimed possible hazard to health, we have included their use as a calorie-lowering or sugar alternative for diabetics who have been advised to do so for medical reasons. (The American Diabetic Association approved its use for diabetics.)

Sugar, whenever used, is limited or cut to a minimum without jeopardizing flavor or recipe structure. Those who wish to use it in place of fructose or other sweeteners may refer to the Table of Equivalents (p. 288) for the appropriate recipe modification.

We discourage the use of any artificial foods, with only one or two exceptions. Egg substitute is offered as an optional ingredient for those who wish to cut calories, cholesterol, or fat. You may use the commercial type or the home recipe made with egg whites in this book. Nutrient analyses are given for the commercial egg substitute. Sugar-free jams and jellies, homemade or otherwise, do cut calories, so we have included them when appropriate.

Sodium

The job of controlling intake of sodium in a technological society has become near impossible. Sodium is found not only naturally in our foods, but is also "hidden" in processed foods, soft drinks, fast foods, water, and even toothpaste. We all eat more sodium than we realize — about ten to fourteen grams per day (equivalent to 2 tablespoons of table salt). And that's more than the U.S. Dietary Goals' recommendation of 8 grams per day. That may mean throwing away the salt shaker. (It also may mean doing away with such salty treats as potato chips, which at 230 mg sodium per ounce can add up, and even such luxuries as some mineral waters, which may contain from 2 mg to 2000 mg sodium parts per million.)

That's why you will not find any salt in the *Light Style* recipes. Instead, we enhance flavors with spices, herbs, fruit juices, fruits, peels, and wine. We think you will be pleasantly surprised with the flavor results of our low-sodium recipes. In fact, if you are a heavy salter, start now to deprogram your taste buds for salt by gradually decreasing the amount used in cooking or at the table until none is used. Studies have shown that the taste buds of high-frequency salters can be "debriefed" within a few months.

We have also included recipes for a number of condiments, such as catsup, baking powder, mustard, and numerous salad dressings, as well as stocks and sauces, that put the sodium and quality controls in the cook's hands. Making your own saves money, too.

The Nutrient Counter beginning on page 266 gives sodium counts for commonly used foods. It can be a valuable guide for controlling sodium in your diet and help you make wise food choices.

Fats

The raging controversy over fat has yet to be resolved. So far there is no conclusive proof that fat—any kind—is responsible for heart disease, cancer, or other killer diseases. Until more is known about this highly complex nutrient, the word is "moderation." Limit total fats and try to distribute the types of fats you eat—saturated animal fat, monounsaturated/polyunsaturated fats—evenly in your diet. This means that the diet should favor fats from vegetable rather than animal sources.

Light Style recipes reduce total fat content in several ways. We emphasize foods that are naturally low in fat, such as fish, shellfish, poultry (without skin), as well as fruits and vegetables, which rarely contain any fat at all. Foods high in fats, such as pork, lamb, ham, and sausage meats, are played down.

We employ calorie-lowering cooking methods, such as steaming, poaching, broiling, baking, grilling, and light sautéing with minimal amounts of fats and encourage the use of nonstick pans. Portion control is another tool for reducing total fat calories, and our recipes help you learn how to do it.

Cutting down on fat wherever possible automatically cuts calories, cholesterol, and total fat intake, too.

Cholesterol

The controversy over cholesterol centers around heart disease. Up to now, cholesterol was believed to be associated with heart attacks. Now studies indicate that the mechanism that transports the fatty substance called cholesterol is the crucial factor in raising or lowering the build-up of plaque. Some people have better ability to move cholesterol out of the body than others. Those who do not (characterized as having too much low-density lipoprotein) have a tendency to develop heart disease. The higher the density of lipoproteins, the less chance of heart attacks. Although dietary cholesterol may not be an important consideration with people with high-density lipoproteins, excessive cholesterol intake could adversely affect people who are prone to heart problems. Diet is only one way such people can create favorable high-density lipoproteins (HDL) levels. Factors such as lack of exercise, heavy use of tobacco, exposure to other pollutants, and family history may also have a lot to do with susceptibility to heart disease. (Studies also show that vigorously active individuals and people with family histories of longevity have higher levels of HDLs and develop fewer heart attacks than others.)

For those who must and should reduce cholesterol intake, *Light Style* recipes provide several options. Vegetable oils and margarines that contain no cholesterol are given in the recipes. All the recipes, in fact, include cholesterol counts. The Nutrient Counter (p. 266), too, has cholesterol counts for commonly used foods.

You can lower intake of cholesterol, too, by simply reducing total calories if you are overweight. Limit foods high in cholesterol such as organ meats, highly marbled beef, sausages, cold cuts, some shellfish, butter and eggs. Discard excess fat from stews and sauces using meats high in animal fats, and use nonfat milk and milk products.

For those who must watch cholesterol, egg yolks should be limited. We provide recipes using egg substitute for such individuals. If they pose no problem, eggs are an excellent source of high quality inexpensive protein and are easy to digest. They contain more nutrients per volume than any other natural food and are a fine choice for meals within moderation, especially for the elderly on fixed incomes.

The Recipes

There are over 250 recipes that are not only low in calories, fat, cholesterol, and salt, but serve as a valuable guide for light eating that comes from knowledge. The recipes are not only delicious, but they also teach you how to modify them to suit your personal needs.

All the recipes have been tested several times and under several conditions. They have been tested at hospitals, restaurants, and homes. They have been prepared by experienced chefs and by home cooks who have never cooked before. We have given the recipes a final home-test to make sure that even the novice cook finds them foolproof.

In *Light Style*, you will find fancy and everyday recipes, dozens of appetizers, soups, stocks, breads, eggs, crêpes, fish and shellfish, poultry, game, meats, pastas and rice, vegetables, salads, salad dressings, sauces, condiments, desserts, and beverages.

All of the recipes include nutrient calculations for calories, fats, cholesterol, and sodium. The calculations are based on nutrient values found in several authoritative sources: "Composition of Foods," Agriculture Handbooks No. 8 and 456 (Agricultural Research Service, USDA); *Food Values of Portions Commonly Used*, Bowes and Church (J. B. Lippincott Company); *Dictionary of Calories and Carbohydrates*, Barbara Kraus (Grosset & Dunlap); and *The Dictionary of Sodium, Fats, and Cholesterol*, by Barbara Kraus (Grosset & Dunlap). The calculations were done by four dietitians to assure accuracy.

All nutrient analyses after each recipe are based on the ingredients listed. When more than one choice is given, the nutrient analysis will favor the first choice. For instance, a recipe calling for "egg substitute or eggs," will contain the Nutrient Analysis for the egg substitute. Check the Nutrient Counter if you wish to adjust the nutrient count to the second-choice ingredient.

Because no two source books listing nutrient values of foods contain identical nutrient counts of the individual foods, a variance of 10% to 15% in values may occur.

Most of the recipes contain roughly half the calories, fat, and sodium found in comparable dishes. Basic cooking recommendations also have been added for those who need them. All have been simplified to make use of the most basic home equipment.

Special Recipes

Staple recipes, which can be made at home at a fraction of the cost of the commercial types, are also given. Low-sodium, low-calorie, low-cholesterol, and low-fat sauces, stocks, catsup, egg substitute, mustard and salad dressings are valuable additions to any health-minded cook's repertoire.

Menus

Having a party? Calling the neighbors in for Sunday TV football lunch? Going Mexican, Italian, or Chinese tonight? The menus with nutrient counts will help you plan any occasion.

Modifying Recipes

You will find tips for substituting sweetening agents, eggs, salt, flavorings, fats, and creams. The tips will help you modify any recipe to suit your individual dietary need.

Daily Food Guide

The guide is based on the United States Department of Agriculture recommendations for serving sizes considered nutritionally adequate for adults, children, and pregnant women. It will help you plan menus based on balanced food concepts. You can be sure that by following the Basic Four Food Group serving-size recommendation, you will be providing your body with a safe margin of baseline nutrients needed for fitness and good health.

Weight Control

Maintaining ideal body weight is the best preventive health tool anyone can employ to reduce intake of fat, cholesterol, sugar, and salt in your diet. There is a chapter on the importance of maintaining ideal weight and ways to achieve it.

Nutrient Counter

The Nutrient Counter lists calories, sodium, fat, and cholesterol contents of commonly used foods in household measures. We have separated the listings for beef, veal, pork, lamb, fish, shellfish, and cheese for easier reference.

Alcohol Exchange List

The list of commonly used alcoholic beverages gives the calorie-watcher and the diabetic who must calculate alcohol calories in their diet a graphic look at some of these calories.

Spice and Herb Chart

The chart is designed to help the cook learn how to enhance the flavors of meat, fish, poultry, sauces, soups, vegetables, seafood, and baked goods without using salt. We hope the guide will inspire an adventuresome spirit.

Table of Substitutions

The value of this chart is to make you a better evaluator and adapter of recipes, ingredients, and nutrients. You'll find the measure of equivalents of artificial and natural sweeteners and other commonly used ingredients for quick and easy reference.

Table of Measurement Equivalents

The table of liquid and solid measures in both standard and metric units will help you make conversions.

Meat Thermometer

The graphic "thermometer" tells you when poultry, lamb, pork, veal, and beef are done.

Special Products

The list of special brand name products used in the book includes a brief description of the product, where to find it, and our evaluation of it.

Glossary

We have included definitions for some of the nutritional terms used in this book.

We invite you to treat this book as a handbook for recipe modification and meal planning. The tools are provided: the recipes; the scientifically based nutrient analysis of each recipe that will help you plan menus and control nutrient intake; and the charts that will help you substitute ingredients or modify recipes. We have provided tips for experimenting with herbs, spices, and wines, improving the nutritional quality of appetizers, and creating your own supply of pantry-shelf condiments, sauces, and dressings. The book provides information about servings and stresses the importance of portion control for sound nutrition and weight control.

If calories are a concern, the recipes will show you how to reduce them. Anyone who needs to cut salt intake will find an exciting array of low-sodium recipes that will drive away any sense of deprivation. If fat or cholesterol intake is a problem (or even if it's not but you want to lower them anyway), the recipes automatically do it for you, and charts and tables show you how your own recipes can be lowered as well. You'll make most efficient use of the book if you read the chapter introductions and familiarize yourself with its content.

The relationship between the recipes and the nutritional information provided in every chapter will, we hope, make you more knowledgeable about food choices.

Most of all, we hope the book will prove that low-calorie, low-fat, low-salt eating can also be high in flavor appeal.

Appetizers

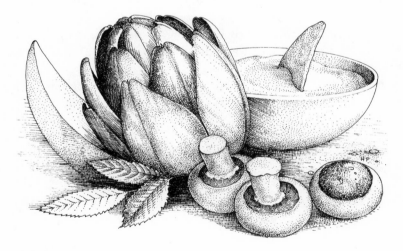

$\mathcal{T}$here is no need to avoid appetizers or treat them as empty calories that make you fat, if you bank them into your total daily nutrition account.

Some wise mothers we know work fruits, vegetables, and dairy products into family meals through appetizers, especially when there are growing children who might not get enough of them at meal times.

A wise cocktail party hostess, too, plans a variety of appetizers from all four food groups, especially for holiday revellers and single men and women who may miss a regular meal that day. She serves a fruit and vegetable tray with yogurt or cheese dips, some meat, fish, or poultry in the form of teriyaki or meatballs, whole grains in the form of crackers, bread, or toast. It's easy to accrue a balanced meal by the end of that party!

We have tried to keep total calories, salt, and fat down while maintaining high nutrient density in our collection of appetizers. Each and every appetizer given will make some nutritional contribution to your total daily food intake.

Here's how you can do it, using *Light Style:*

- Avoid frying foods or using excess fat. Fats provide more calories per volume than any other nutrient.
- Emphasize fruits and vegetables. They contain fewer calories than foods containing sugars, starches, and even meats and dairy products.
- Trim off excess fat from meats and use lean meats whenever possible. (Chicken and fish have fewer calories than red meat.)
- Eliminate salt and replace with complementary herbs and spices.
- Reduce cholesterol by using polyunsaturated oils (vegetable

oils lowest in hydrogenated fats, such as corn oil, safflower oil, soy, and cottonseed oils).
• Practice portion control.

You'll find an exciting array of appetizers that will suit most any party situation, from the elbow-to-elbow party-time goodies to the elegant sit-down dinner appetizers. Many of the appetizers, such as the meatballs, pizza, and dips, can be made well in advance and stored either in the freezer or refrigerator until ready to use.

CRAB DIP

1 pound cooked crab meat (fresh or frozen)
1 cup low-fat cottage cheese
2 tablespoons low-sodium, low-calorie
  Mayonnaise (p. 200)
1 tablespoon Dijon Mustard (p. 203)
1 tablespoon fresh lemon juice
Thin lemon slices, twisted
Parsley sprigs

Combine crab meat, cottage cheese, mayonnaise, mustard, and lemon juice in a blender container and blend until smooth. Serve garnished with twists of lemon and parsley sprigs. Makes 2 cups.

NOTE: Canned crab has a very high sodium content. We suggest that those watching their salt intake use only fresh or frozen Alaskan king crab meat.

Each 1 tablespoon serving contains about:
  25 calories
  32 mg sodium (content unavailable for crab)
  13 g fat
  15 mg cholesterol
  Exchanges: ½ meat

GUACAMOLE

1 large avocado
2 tablespoons fresh lemon juice
1 clove garlic, minced
1 small tomato, peeled and chopped
2 green onions, chopped
¼ green bell pepper, minced, or
    ½ teaspoon chopped green chile pepper
½ teaspoon chili powder
1 tablespoon minced cilantro (fresh coriander)
Pepper to taste

Cut avocado in half and remove pit. Scoop out pulp into a bowl and mash with a fork. Add lemon juice, garlic, tomato, green onions, green pepper, chili powder, cilantro, and pepper and mix well. Makes about 1¼ cups.

Each 1 tablespoon serving contains about:
28 calories
1 mg sodium
2 g fat
0 mg cholesterol
Exchanges: ½ fat

SEAFOOD DIP

½ cup low-calorie sour cream
½ cup low-fat plain yogurt
½ cup shredded cooked crab meat (fresh or frozen)
¼ teaspoon Worcestershire sauce
2 cloves garlic, minced
3 tablespoons fresh lemon juice

Combine sour cream, yogurt, crab meat, Worcestershire sauce, garlic, and lemon juice and mix well. Serve with cut raw vegetables, such as carrots, zucchini, jicama, green and red peppers, snow peas, and green beans. Makes about 1½ cups.

NOTE: Canned crab has a very high sodium content. We suggest that those watching their salt intake use only fresh or frozen Alaskan king crab meat.

Each 2 tablespoon serving contains about:
  24 calories
  12 mg sodium (content unavailable for crab)
  3 g fat
  5 mg cholesterol
  Exchanges: ¼ meat

SKINNY DIP

  ½ cup low-sodium, low-calorie Mayonnaise (p. 200)
1½ cups low-fat plain yogurt
  4 green onions, chopped
  3 tablespoons fresh lemon juice
  2 cloves garlic, minced
  1 (10-ounce) package frozen chopped spinach,
      thawed, drained, and squeezed dry

Combine mayonnaise, yogurt, onion, lemon juice, and garlic. Let stand 30 minutes, to allow flavors to blend. Fold in spinach. Serve with cut raw vegetables, such as carrots, cauliflowerets, zucchini, celery, green or red bell peppers, jicama, and green beans. Makes 2½ cups.

Each 1 tablespoon serving contains about:
  26 calories
  15 mg sodium
  3 g fat
  3 mg cholesterol
  Exchanges: ½ fat

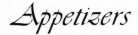

APPETIZER ARTICHOKES

6 large artichokes
Water
2 tablespoons coriander seeds
Juice of 2 lemons
Curry Mayonnaise (p. 201), Drawn Margarine (p. 189),
    Vinaigrette (p. 182)

Trim rough outer leaves from artichokes. Cut stems even with bottoms. Place artichokes upright in a pan in which they fit snugly. Add water to cover, coriander seeds, and lemon juice and bring to a boil. Reduce to a simmer, cover, and cook until outer leaves pull off easily, about 40 minutes. Let cool. Hold cooked artichokes upright under a steady stream of cold water. Leaves will open out, exposing choke and center leaves. Pull out center leaves with fingers. Using a spoon, scrape out remaining choke fibers and small leaves. Fill centers with 2 tablespoons Curry Mayonnaise, or chill and serve with Drawn Margarine or Vinaigrette. Makes 6 servings.

    1 artichoke without sauce contains about:
    44 calories
    30 mg sodium
    0 g fat
    0 mg cholesterol
    Exchanges: 1 B vegetable

CHAMPAGNE MEATBALLS

1 pound lean ground beef sirloin
Freshly ground pepper to taste
1 tablespoon minced onion
1 teaspoon minced garlic
1 tablespoon egg substitute, or
    1 small egg, lightly beaten
½ cup low-calorie grape jelly
¼ cup Catsup (p. 203)
½ cup Champagne or dry white wine

In a mixing bowl, mix together beef, pepper, onion, garlic, and egg substitute or egg. Form mixture into 36 (1-inch) balls, set aside. In a skillet, combine grape jelly, Catsup, and Champagne and simmer, uncovered, 5 minutes to blend flavors. Add meatballs and simmer, uncovered, 30 minutes, stirring often. Makes 36 meatballs.

NOTE: Meatballs may be stored in the freezer before or after cooking. To cook from raw frozen state, thaw slightly, then cook as directed. To heat from cooked frozen state, thaw slightly and place in a 350°F oven about 15 minutes, or until heated through.

Each meatball contains about:
   30 calories
   15 mg sodium
   2 g fat
   12 mg cholesterol
   Exchanges: ¼ meat

CHICKEN PACIFICA

1 tablespoon Low-Calorie Margarine (p. 207)
½ cup Low-Calorie Russian Dressing (p. 183)
1½ tablespoons low-calorie apricot jelly
3 whole chicken breasts, skinned, boned,
    and cut in 1-inch cubes

In a small saucepan, melt margarine over low heat. Add dressing and apricot jelly and blend thoroughly. Heat through. Place chicken cubes in a baking dish and cover with dressing-jelly mixture. Marinate chicken, refrigerated, 3 to 6 hours. One hour before cooking, remove chicken from refrigerator and allow to come to room temperature. Leave chicken in pan used for marinating and place in a 350°F oven for 20 minutes, or until lightly browned. Remove meat from marinade and serve with wood picks. Makes about 50 pieces.

Each piece contains about:
17 calories
13 mg sodium
trace fat
7 mg cholesterol
Exchanges: ⅛ meat

MELON WITH PORT

This can double as a dessert.

1 large honeydew or melon of choice
½ cup port wine
Fresh mint sprigs

Cut melon in half, remove and discard seeds. Using a melon scoop, carve balls from melon flesh and place them in a bowl. Pour wine over melon balls and chill several hours for flavors to blend. Serve in sherbet dishes and garnish with mint sprigs. Makes 6 servings.

Each ½ cup serving contains about:
50 calories
40 mg sodium
0 g fat
0 mg cholesterol
Exchanges: 1 fruit

PIZZA

1 envelope active dry yeast
¾ cup lukewarm water (105° to 115°F)
½ teaspoon fructose
2 cups sifted unbleached flour
1½ teaspoons vegetable oil or olive oil
1 tablespoon yellow cornmeal
1 cup Italian Meat Sauce (p. 192)
¾ cup shredded mozzarella cheese
½ cup sliced mushrooms
½ onion, sliced in rings
½ green bell pepper, sliced in rings
½ red bell pepper, sliced in rings
1½ tablespoons grated Parmesan cheese (optional)

Dissolve yeast in lukewarm water. Add fructose and let yeast mixture stand 10 minutes. Measure flour into a mixing bowl. Add yeast mixture and stir in thoroughly. On a lightly floured board, knead about 5 minutes, or until soft and pliable. Form dough into ball and place in a lightly greased bowl. Turn ball to grease top, cover bowl, and let rise in a warm place about 2 hours, or until doubled in bulk.

Grease a 14-inch pizza pan or 11-by-17-inch baking sheet with ½ teaspoon of the oil. Sprinkle pan evenly with cornmeal. Punch down dough and roll out on a lightly floured board into a 14-inch circle to fit pizza pan or a rectangle to fit baking sheet. Place dough in pan and pat and stretch it to fit the pan, pinching up a rim around the edges. Pierce dough in several places with a fork. Spread Italian Meat Sauce over the crust and let it rest about 10 minutes. (At this point, pizza may be frozen for up to 1 week; thaw before proceeding with recipe.) Cover crust with a layer of mozzarella cheese. Arrange mushrooms, onions, and green and red peppers over cheese. Brush vegetables with remaining teaspoon of oil. Sprinkle with Parmesan cheese. Bake at 450°F about 25 minutes, or until browned. Serve at once. Cut into 8 portions. Makes 8 servings.

Each serving with Parmesan cheese contains about:
150 calories
182 mg sodium
3 g fat
12 mg cholesterol
Exchanges: 1 bread, ½ meat, 1 vegetable

Pizza Canapes

Prepare dough as directed for Pizza. Divide dough into 14 portions. Roll each portion into a circle about 2 inches in diameter. Place canapes on baking sheet and top as directed in recipe. Bake at 450°F for 15 minutes.

Each canape with Parmesan cheese contains about:
75 calories
91 mg sodium
1 g fat
6 mg cholesterol
Exchanges: 1 bread, ¼ meat, ½ vegetable

SCALLOPS DEJONGHE

This dish is high in sodium, so beware if you are on a sodium-restricted diet.

2 tablespoons Low-Calorie Margarine (p. 207)
2 cloves garlic, minced
1 cup soft French Bread (p. 49) crumbs without crust
1½ pounds scallops or cleaned shrimp
1 tablespoons sweet Marsala wine
Lemon wedges
Parsley sprigs

In a mixing bowl, cream margarine with garlic. Add crumbs, stirring well to form a paste. Place scallops in 6 individual scallop shells or flameproof ramekins or in a nonstick baking pan. Spread crumb mixture over scallops. Sprinkle with Marsala and broil 4 inches from source of heat until browned, about 10 minutes. Garnish with lemon wedges and parsley sprigs. Makes 6 servings.

Each 4 ounce serving contains about:
133 calories
347 mg sodium
2 g fat
40 mg cholesterol
Exchanges: 3 meat, ¼ bread

SEAFOOD COCKTAIL

**½ pound *each* cooked lobster meat, crab meat, and
    cleaned shrimp (about 12)**
Seafood Cocktail Sauce (p. 208)
Lemon wedges

Cut lobster and crab into 1-inch pieces. Arrange lobster, crab, and
shrimp on a serving platter or on a bed of shaved ice. Serve with Seafood Cocktail Sauce and garnish with lemon wedges. Makes 6
servings.

  Each serving lobster (2 pieces) without sauce contains about:
    30 calories
    30 mg sodium
    trace fat
    12 mg cholesterol
    Exchanges: ¼ meat

  Each serving crab meat (2 pieces) without sauce contains about:
    26 calories
    Sodium figures unavailable for crab
    trace fat
    15 mg cholesterol
    Exchanges: ¼ meat

  Each serving shrimp (2 pieces) without sauce contains about:
    36 calories
    30 mg sodium
    trace fat
    20 mg cholesterol
    Exchanges: ¼ meat

SIRLOIN TERIYAKI

1 pound top beef sirloin, cut in ½-inch cubes
**1 (10½-ounce) can water-packed mandarin orange
    sections, drained**
¾ cup Soy Sauce (p. 209)

Thread sirloin cubes on 12 presoaked bamboo skewers or small metal skewers alternately with mandarin orange sections. Arrange in a single layer in a shallow dish. Pour Soy Sauce over skewers and marinate, refrigerated, 1 hour. Place under broiler or on a barbecue grill and cook to desired doneness. Makes 12 servings.

Each skewer contains about:
65 calories
15 mg sodium
5 g fat
20 mg cholesterol
Exchanges: 1 meat

STUFFED MUSHROOMS

12 large mushrooms (1½ to 2 inches in diameter)
¾ pound lean ground beef sirloin
2 cloves garlic, minced
¼ cup fresh lemon juice
¼ teaspoon pepper
Pinch dried thyme
1 bay leaf
1½ teaspoons ground coriander
2½ teaspoons chopped cilantro (fresh coriander)
1½ teaspoons low-calorie margarine
⅛ teaspoon paprika
½ cup dry white wine

Remove stems from mushrooms. Set caps aside and chop stems. In a skillet, combine meat, chopped stems, and garlic and cook over medium heat until meat is browned and crumbly. Add lemon juice, pepper, thyme, bay leaf, coriander, and cilantro. Cook until flavors are blended, about 5 minutes.

While meat mixture is cooking, melt margarine in a skillet and add paprika, wine, and mushroom caps. Cover and cook over medium heat until mushrooms are just tender, about 7 minutes. Stuff caps with meat mixture and place on a greased baking sheet. Broil 2 inches from source of heat 5 minutes or until golden. Makes 12 servings.

Each stuffed mushroom contains about:
30 calories
12 mg sodium
2 g fat
13 mg cholesterol
Exchanges: ½ meat

STUFFED CHERRY TOMATOES

1½ cups Cream Cheese (p. 208)
¼ cup grated carrot
¼ cup finely chopped celery
2 tablespoons finely chopped green bell pepper
2 tablespoons finely chopped red bell pepper
¾ teaspoon Herb Blend (p. 206)
Pinch garlic powder
Dash hot pepper sauce
48 cherry tomatoes
2 tablespoons sesame seeds, toasted*

Combine Cream Cheese, carrot, celery, green and red peppers, Herb Blend, garlic powder, and hot pepper sauce in a bowl. Stir until well mixed. Cut a shallow slice off stem end of each cherry tomato. Remove seeds and pulp, leaving shells intact. Fill each tomato shell with a teaspoonful of cheese mixture. Sprinkle with sesame seeds. Makes 48 stuffed tomatoes.

* To toast sesame seeds, place in a dry pan over medium heat and heat, shaking pan gently, until golden.

Each stuffed tomato contains about:
15 calories
18 mg sodium
1 g fat
2 mg cholesterol
Exchanges: ¼ B vegetable

TORTILLA SALAD

  6 corn tortillas
1½ tablespoons safflower oil
  3 tablespoons red wine vinegar
  2 tablespoons chopped cilantro (fresh coriander)
  1 small sweet white onion, chopped
  1 large tomato, diced
  ½ avocado, diced (optional)

Cut each tortilla into 4 triangular pieces. Place the tortilla triangles on a baking sheet and put under the broiler for about 1 minute on each side, or until crisp. In a bowl, combine oil, vinegar, and cilantro. Add tortillas, onion, tomato, and avocado, if desired, and toss to coat well. Makes 6 servings.

Each serving with avocado contains about:
    114 calories
    3 mg sodium
    7 g fat
    0 mg cholesterol
    Exchanges: 1 bread, 1 fat

Each serving without avocado contains about:
    83 calories
    3 mg sodium
    4 g fat
    0 mg cholesterol
    Exchanges: ½ bread, ½ fat

Soups and Stocks

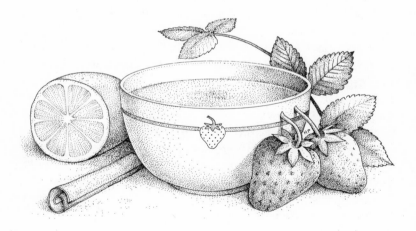

$\mathcal{T}$here are several advantages to making your own stocks and soups. You'll find, first of all, that your own homemade batch is far superior in flavor to most any commercial types on the supermarket shelf. Making your own soups and stocks will also remove the guesswork and worry over preservatives, excess fat, and salt content often found in commercial brands. And, of course, the cost of homemade stocks and soups beats most found in a can, salted or not!

A saltless soup or stock, however, needs all the help it can get from the herb and spice department. You will probably learn more about blending flavors here than in any other chapter. You may even become your own herb and spice specialist and discover exciting flavor combinations.

Set aside ample time for cooking stocks and be prepared to store them properly in the refrigerator. You will need a few extra-large pots to cook large quantities at a time and large jars with tight-fitting lids for storage. You will always want to have stock on hand for steaming vegetables, cooking pasta and rice, and making sauces, for they provide flavor to foods prepared without salt.

We also suggest freezing the stocks in pint-size freezer containers for convenient handling when large quantities of stocks are called for, or in ice-cube trays when stocks are used only as a seasoning in a sauce.

You can store stocks or soups safely up to a week in the refrigerator or four months in the freezer.

Soups are relatively low in calories and can be made high in nutrients with a few simple additions of vegetable or meat. A basic vegetable soup, for instance, can be transformed into a meal-in-a-dish with the addition of beans, meat, or poultry. Add some rice, macaroni, or barley and the soup is enriched. A robust whole-meal soup can be a wonderfully nourishing supper, often needing nothing more than some bread and a salad to round out the meal.

You'll find the calorie content of these soups relatively low. And the tricks we use can easily be adapted to your own recipes. We use arrowroot or cornstarch in place of flour for a lower-caloried thickener. It's not that arrowroot or cornstarch contains fewer calories than flour. Less is needed to thicken the sauce; ergo, the fewer calories you consume.

Fats are used minimally and trimmed whenever possible. The type of fat you choose could affect cholesterol count, so if cholesterol is a concern use the recommended polyunsaturated fat and skim milk or trim any animal fat. An easy way to rid the soup or stock of animal or hydrogenated fat is to chill it long enough to coagulate the fat on the surface, then skim it off.

Hot Soups

ALBONDIGAS SOUP

   1 pound ground lean beef
  ½ teaspoon pepper
   2 tablespoons chopped parsley
   2 cloves garlic, minced
   1 tablespoon egg substitute, or 1 small egg, beaten
   4 tablespoons chopped cilantro (fresh coriander)
   1 teaspoon dried oregano
   3 tablespoons long-grain rice
   1 small onion, minced
   1 teaspoon vegetable oil
1½ quarts low-sodium Beef Stock (p. 39)
   1 cup peeled and diced tomatoes, preferably
      Italian plum
   6 medium carrots, sliced
   2 cups sliced celery
   1 cup corn kernels (fresh or frozen only)

Combine ground beef, pepper, parsley, garlic, egg substitute or egg, 1 tablespoon of the cilantro, oregano, and rice. Form into meatballs about 1 inch in diameter; set aside.

In a large saucepan, sauté the onion in oil until tender. Add stock and tomatoes and bring to a boil. Add carrots and celery. Drop meatballs into boiling stock. Add corn, reduce heat to low, cover, and simmer 30 minutes. Stir in remaining cilantro and serve. Makes 8 servings.

Each 1 cup serving contains about:
176 calories
108 mg sodium
4 g fat
53 mg cholesterol
Exchanges: 1 meat, 1 B vegetable

CHICKEN SOUP KLARA

⅓ bunch parsley
½ bunch dill
Tops of 2 parsley roots
1 pound chicken pieces
3 leeks, cut in ½-inch pieces
1 onion, cut in wedges
1 clove garlic, minced
3 parsley roots, peeled and diced
4 carrots, cut in halves
3 stalks celery, sliced
2 quarts low-sodium Chicken Stock (p. 40)

Tie parsley, dill, and parsley root tops into a bouquet garni. Place in a large kettle with chicken, leeks, onion, garlic, parsley roots, carrots, celery, and stock. Bring to a boil, reduce heat, and simmer, partially covered, over low heat 1½ hours, removing froth from surface as needed. Discard bouquet garni. Chill soup until fat coagulates on surface, then lift off fat. Skin and bone chicken pieces, cut meat into cubes and return to pot. Reheat to serving temperature. Makes 16 servings.

Each ½ cup serving contains about:
44 calories
16 mg sodium
2 g fat
23 mg cholesterol
Exchanges: ½ meat, ½ vegetable

CHINATOWN SOUP

1½ quarts low-sodium Chicken Stock (p. 40)
2 cups firmly packed coarsely chopped spinach
¼ cup chopped green onion
1 teaspoon minced ginger root
½ cup julienne-cut cooked pork roast
⅛ teaspoon white pepper
4 ounces cooked crab meat, lobster meat, or
    chicken breast meat, diced
1 egg white, lightly beaten
1 teaspoon cornstarch
1 tablespoon water

Bring chicken stock to a boil. Add spinach and return to a boil. Reduce heat and simmer 1 minute. Add green onions, ginger, pork, and pepper and simmer 2 to 3 minutes longer. Add meat of choice and heat through. Add egg white to simmering soup in a slow, steady stream and cook until egg white sets. Mix cornstarch with water until smooth and stir into soup. Cook and stir until soup is transparent. Serve at once. Makes 6 servings.

Each 1 cup serving contains about:
31 calories
39 mg sodium
1 g fat
17 mg cholesterol
Exchanges: ½ meat, 1 vegetable

CONSOMME MADRILENE

1 cup *each* thinly sliced celery, leeks, and carrots
3 cups whole peeled tomatoes
1 teaspoon dried thyme
½ bay leaf
1 sprig parsley
1 green bell pepper, sliced
¼ cup sliced canned pimiento, drained
8 peppercorns
¼ cup dry Sherry
½ cup thinly sliced turnip
2 quarts low-sodium Beef Stock (p. 39)
2 egg whites, beaten
White pepper to taste (optional)

Combine celery, leeks, carrots, tomatoes, thyme, bay leaf, parsley, green pepper, pimiento, peppercorns, Sherry, and turnip in a large saucepan. Add stock and egg whites. Bring to a boil, reduce heat, cover, and simmer for 1½ hours; do not allow to boil. Strain through fine cheesecloth into a bowl. Add pepper to taste. Consommé should be clear. Makes 8 servings.

Each 1 cup serving contains about:
16 calories
18 mg sodium
trace fat
2 mg cholesterol
Exchanges: negligible

FRENCH ONION SOUP

   1 tablespoon low-calorie margarine
   6 medium onions, thinly sliced
   ¼ teaspoon fructose
   1 tablespoon arrowroot
   2 tablespoons water
   2 quarts low-sodium Beef Stock, heated (p. 39)
   ½ cup dry white wine
   Pepper to taste
1½ tablespoons Cognac (optional)
   1 tablespoon grated Parmesan cheese (optional)

Melt margarine in a saucepan. Add onions and fructose, cover, and cook over low heat 15 minutes. Uncover, increase heat to medium and cook, stirring frequently, until onions are tender and golden, about 40 minutes. Dissolve arrowroot in water and add to pan with stock. Bring to a boil, then reduce heat to a simmer. Add wine and pepper, partially cover, and cook for 30 minutes. When ready to serve, stir in Cognac and sprinkle with Parmesan cheese, if desired. Makes 8 servings.

   Each 1 cup serving with cheese contains about:
   56 calories
   64 mg sodium
   1 g fat
   1 mg cholesterol
   Exchanges: 1 B vegetable

HEARTY MINESTRONE

The next day, add some leftover meat and you've got a nutritious meal-in-a-dish.

>   ½ cup Great Northern beans, soaked overnight in
>   water and drained
>   1 tablespoon olive oil
>   1 clove garlic, minced
>   1 cup thinly sliced onions
>   1 cup diced carrots
>   1 cup diced celery
>   ½ cup diced peeled potatoes
>   2 cups diced zucchini
>   1 cup diced green beans
>   3 cups shredded cabbage
>   1½ quarts low-sodium Beef Stock (p. 39)
>   4 Italian plum tomatoes, peeled, or
>   1 (8-ounce) can low-sodium canned tomatoes,
>   with their liquid
>   1 teaspoon dried basil
>   ½ cup elbow macaroni
>   ¼ cup freshly grated Parmesan cheese (optional)

Put beans in a saucepan and add water to cover by 2 inches. Bring to a moderate boil, cover, and cook until beans are tender, about 40 minutes. Let stand in cooking liquid until ready to use.

While beans are cooking, heat oil in a large kettle. Add garlic and onions and cook over medium heat until the onions are tender and golden but not browned. Add the carrots and cook, stirring frequently, for 3 minutes. Repeat this procedure with the celery, potato, zucchini, and green beans, cooking each vegetable for 3 minutes. Add the cabbage. Cook, stirring occasionally, about 5 minutes. Add stock, tomatoes with their liquid, and basil. Cover and simmer for at least 3 hours.

About 15 minutes before the soup is done, drain beans and add with macaroni to soup. Just before removing from heat, swirl in Parmesan cheese if desired. Makes 10 servings.

Each ½ cup serving without Parmesan cheese contains about:
56 calories
7 mg sodium

trace fat
trace cholesterol
Exchanges: 1 B vegetable

LOBSTER BISQUE

1 small carrot, sliced
1 medium onion, chopped
2 peppercorns
1 bay leaf
Pinch dried thyme
1 sprig parsley
6 cups Fish Stock (p. 41)
¾ cup dry white wine
1 pound uncooked small lobster tails
½ cup low-calorie margarine
3 tablespoons arrowroot
1 cup nonfat milk
1 cup evaporated nonfat milk
2 tablespoons dry Sherry
Paprika

Combine carrot, onion, peppercorns, bay leaf, thyme, parsley, and stock in a 4-quart saucepan. Bring to a boil, add wine and lobster, reduce heat, and simmer 10 minutes. Remove lobster tails. Continue simmering cooking liquid 35 minutes, then strain through a fine sieve and set aside. When lobster tails are cool enough to handle, remove meat from shells and dice coarsely; set aside.

Melt margarine in the same saucepan and stir in arrowroot until smooth. Gradually add strained cooking liquid. Bring to a boil, reduce heat, and simmer 10 minutes. Gradually stir in milks and Sherry. Add reserved lobster meat and heat through. Sprinkle with paprika. Makes 10 servings.

Each ½ cup serving contains about:
100 calories
111 mg sodium
7 g fat
41 g cholesterol
Exchanges: 1 meat

PEA SOUP

1 pound green split peas
4 tablespoons low-calorie margarine
4 leeks, coarsely chopped
1 quart water
Bouquet Garni (p. 202)
White pepper to taste
Heart of small head Boston or
    butter lettuce, shredded
7 tablespoons evaporated nonfat milk
1 tablespoon finely chopped parsley
1½ tablespoons dry Sherry
Parsley sprigs

Soak peas in warm water to cover 2 hours. Drain and set aside. Melt margarine in a large saucepan and sauté leeks about 15 minutes, or until tender. Add peas, water, Bouquet Garni, and pepper and bring to a simmer. Cover and cook 1 to 1½ hours, or until peas are tender. Drain and reserve liquid and purée vegetables. Return puréed vegetables and liquid to pot and bring to a boil. Add lettuce and cook 1 minute. Remove from heat and stir in milk, parsley, and Sherry. Return to heat and bring to a gentle simmer. Garnish with parsley sprigs. Makes 8 servings.

Each ½ cup serving contains about:
  80 calories
  94 mg sodium
  3 g fat
  1 mg cholesterol
  Exchanges: 1 meat

POTATO AND LEEK SOUP

   1 tablespoon low-calorie margarine
   4 leeks, cut in ½-inch slices
   1 onion, diced
   4 potatoes, peeled and diced
   4 cups low-sodium Chicken Stock (p. 40)
1½ cups evaporated nonfat milk
  ½ cup nonfat milk
   Pepper to taste

Melt margarine in a large saucepan. Add leeks and onion and cook, covered, until vegetables are tender, stirring occasionally. Add potatoes and stock and simmer, covered, for 40 minutes. Add milks and heat to serving temperature. Season with pepper. Makes 12 servings.

   NOTE: For a smooth soup, place soup with vegetables in a blender container or food processor and blend until smooth. Return purée to pot and add milks and pepper. Heat just to serving temperature.

   Each ½ cup serving contains about:
   73 calories
   62 mg sodium
   trace fat
   1 mg cholesterol
   Exchanges: 1 bread

VEGETABLE SOUP

7 cups low-sodium Chicken Stock (p. 40)
1 cup low-sodium tomato juice
½ cup thinly sliced cabbage
¼ cup chopped onion
3 medium carrots, chopped
3 leeks, sliced
1 cup chopped celery
¼ cup chopped green bell pepper
1 (10-ounce) can low-sodium tomatoes with their
   liquid, or 3 medium tomatoes, peeled
½ cup lima beans (fresh or frozen)
⅛ teaspoon ground cloves
½ cup shelled peas (fresh or frozen)
½ cup corn kernels (fresh or frozen)

Place chicken stock and tomato juice in a large kettle. Add cabbage, onion, carrots, leeks, celery, green pepper, tomatoes, lima beans, and cloves. Bring to a boil, reduce heat, partially cover, and simmer 45 minutes. Add peas and corn and simmer 15 minutes. Makes 8 servings.

Each 1 cup serving contains about:
65 calories
97 mg sodium
trace fat
2 mg cholesterol
Exchanges: 1 B vegetable

Cold Soups

CHILLED BERRY SOUP

1¾ cups water
½ cup rosé wine
¼ cup fructose
2 tablespoons fresh lemon juice
1 stick cinnamon
4 cups fresh or unsweetened frozen strawberries,
    thawed, or berries of choice
1 teaspoon cornstarch
1 tablespoon water
½ cup evaporated nonfat milk

Combine 1¾ cups water, wine, fructose, lemon juice, and cinnamon stick in a saucepan. Bring to a boil and simmer, uncovered, 15 minutes, stirring occasionally. Meanwhile, rinse, hull, and purée berries. Add puréed berries to wine mixture and simmer 10 minutes, stirring frequently. Remove cinnamon stick. Dissolve cornstarch in 1 tablespoon water and stir into berry mixture. Simmer 2 minutes longer. Remove from heat and let cool. Stir milk into berry mixture. Serve chilled or at room temperature. Makes 8 servings.

Each ½ cup serving contains about:
79 calories
20 mg sodium
0 g fat
1 mg cholesterol
Exchanges: 2 fruit

CHILLED CROOKNECK SOUP

4 crookneck squash, sliced
1 medium carrot, sliced
1 large onion, chopped
1 leek, white part only, chopped
2 cloves garlic, minced
¼ teaspoon ground cumin
¼ teaspoon ground nutmeg
3 cups low-sodium Chicken Stock (p. 40)
Dash hot pepper sauce
2 tablespoons low-fat plain yogurt
Chopped chives

Combine squash, carrot, onion, leek, garlic, cumin, nutmeg, and stock in a large saucepan. Bring to a boil, reduce heat, cover, and simmer 15 minutes until tender (overcooking will discolor vegetable). Add hot pepper sauce. Purée soup in blender. Chill thoroughly. Garnish each serving with 1 teaspoon yogurt and chives. Makes 6 servings.

NOTE: If a thinner soup is desired, add chicken stock to desired consistency.

Each ½ cup serving contains about:
30 calories
23 mg sodium
trace fat
1 mg cholesterol
Exchanges: 1 vegetable

GAZPACHO ANDALUZ

1 large cucumber, peeled, seeded, and cut up
1 small onion, cut up
4 medium tomatoes, peeled and cut up
2 cloves garlic, pressed
1 cup low-sodium Chicken Stock (p. 40)
2 cups low-sodium vegetable cocktail juice
1 tablespoon fresh lemon juice
2 tablespoons red wine vinegar
2 teaspoons Worcestershire sauce
2 tablespoons *each* chopped parsley, onion, cucumber,
    cilantro (fresh coriander), and green bell pepper

Combine cucumber, onion, tomatoes, garlic, stock, juice, lemon juice, vinegar, and Worcestershire sauce in a blender container and blend until coarsely chopped. Cover and chill 1 hour. Place parsley, cilantro, and green pepper in small individual bowls. Place gazpacho in a chilled serving bowl on the table and surround with the condiments. Ladle soup into chilled bowls and let each diner add condiments as desired. Makes 6 servings.

Each ¾ cup serving contains about:
  35 calories
  26 mg sodium
  0 g fat
  1 mg cholesterol
  Exchanges: 1 vegetable

Stocks

BEEF OR VEAL STOCK

2½ pounds beef or veal bones with meat on them
  2 medium carrots, chopped
  2 large onions, chopped
  3 quarts plus 2 cups water
  Bouquet Garni (p. 202)

Brown meat bones in a 400° to 450°F oven for 30 minutes. Transfer to stockpot and add carrots, onions, and water and bring to a boil. Add Bouquet Garni, reduce heat to low, cover partially, and simmer about 5 hours, removing froth from surface as necessary. Add boiling water if liquid evaporates below level of ingredients.

Strain stock through a fine sieve into a bowl and let stand 15 minutes. Carefully remove fat that rises to the surface, or place stock, uncovered, in refrigerator until fat coagulates on top and can be lifted off. Store in tightly covered jar in refrigerator up to 1 week, or freeze up to 4 months. Makes 1½ to 2 quarts.

Each cup stock contains about:
22 calories
18 mg sodium
trace fat
2 mg cholesterol
Exchanges: negligible

CHICKEN OR TURKEY STOCK

3 pounds chicken or turkey bones with meat on them
2 medium carrots, chopped
2 large onions, chopped
3 quarts water
Bouquet Garni (p. 202)

Combine chicken, carrots, onions, and water in a stockpot. Bring to a boil and add Bouquet Garni. Reduce heat to low, cover partially, and simmer about 2 hours, removing froth from surface as necessary. Add boiling water if liquid evaporates below level of ingredients.

Strain stock through a fine sieve into a bowl and let stand 15 minutes. Carefully remove fat that rises to the surface, or place stock, uncovered, in refrigerator until fat coagulates on top and can be lifted off. Store in tightly covered jar in refrigerator up to 1 week, or freeze up to 4 months. Makes 1½ to 2 quarts.

Each cup stock contains about:
26 calories
16 mg sodium
trace fat
trace cholesterol
Exchanges: negligible

FISH STOCK

2 pounds fish bones
1 quart water
2 large onions, chopped
2 sprigs parsley
1 large carrot, chopped
Bouquet Garni (p. 202)

Place fish bones and water in a saucepan and bring to a boil. Add onions, parsley, carrot and Bouquet Garni. Skim any froth that forms on the surface. Reduce heat, partially cover, and simmer 30 minutes. Strain through fine sieve. Store in tightly covered jar in refrigerator up to 1 week, or freeze up to 4 months. Makes 1 quart.

Each ½ cup stock contains about:
15 calories
13 mg sodium
trace fat
trace cholesterol
Exchanges: negligible

Breads

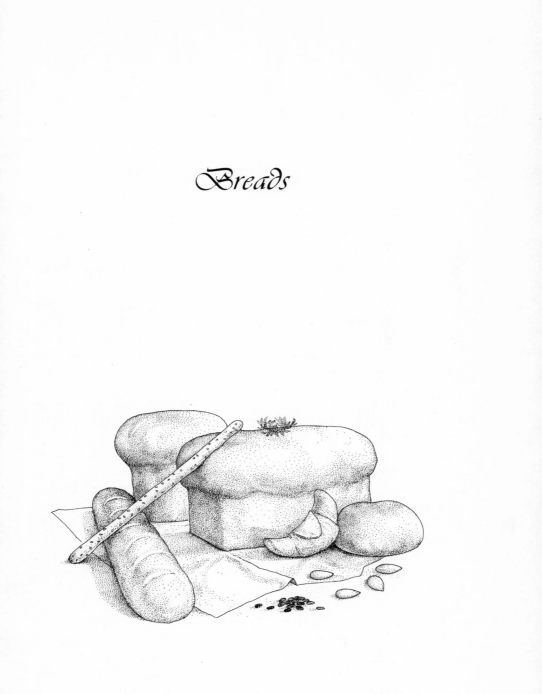

$\mathcal{A}$ common misconception is that bread, a carbohydrate (starch), is fattening. Yet a gram of carbohydrate provides the same calories as protein—4 calories per gram. It's the butter that you add to bread that drives the calories up. (There are 9 calories per gram in fat!)

Bread contributes significant amounts of B vitamins (thiamin, niacin, and riboflavin), iron, plus carbohydrates which the body needs to effectively metabolize nutrients. B vitamins are necessary for maintaining healthy nerves, good muscle tone, healthy skin, and good digestion, among other functions. Iron helps carry oxygen for energy.

Whole-grain breads are also good sources of fiber, which helps promote regular elimination by making the unabsorbed food product in the intestine bulkier and softer.

So does it make sense to drop bread from the diet? Instead, control the size and amount of each portion for weight control. It might help to remember that one serving of bread is only 1 slice or 1 ounce. According to the USDA you will need 4 servings from the grain group, which includes cereals, rice, and other grains, in addition to bread.

All of the bread recipes given here are low in calories, salt, fat, and sugar. In fact, they will be excellent models for modifying your own bread recipes. For instance, when a recipe calls for butter, use low-calorie margarine and save half the fat calories. Substitute fructose in recipes calling for sugar to save at least half the sugar calories. Egg substitute can replace eggs if you are very concerned about reducing calories or need to watch cholesterol intake for medical reasons.

We have found that we can eliminate salt altogether in bread recipes at no cost to flavor. If you are timid about starting to cut salt in your cooking, the bread chapter is a friendly place to start.

Some breads will, incidentally, make wonderful gifts from your kitchen at holiday time. Our favorite is Ramona's Whole Wheat Bread, which has only 70 calories a slice, 30 milligrams sodium, and hardly any fat. It's so rich you won't miss slathering it with butter or anything else. It's almost a dessert in itself!

Novelty Breads

CLOUD BISCUITS

2 cups unbleached flour
2 teaspoons fructose
4 teaspoons low-sodium baking powder
½ cup low-calorie margarine
3 tablespoons egg substitute, or 1 egg, beaten
½ cup nonfat milk

In a large mixing bowl, sift together flour, fructose, and baking powder. With a pastry blender, cut in margarine until the mixture resembles coarse crumbs. Combine egg substitute or egg and milk and add to flour mixture all at once. Stir until dough is just moistened; do not overmix.

Turn dough out on a lightly floured board and knead *gently* with heel of one hand, about 20 strokes in all. Roll dough out ¾-inch thick, flouring board as needed. Dip a 2-inch biscuit cutter in flour and cut straight down through dough without twisting. Repeat until all dough is cut, dipping the cutter in flour each time. Place circles on an ungreased baking sheet ¾ inch apart for crusty biscuits or close together for ones with soft sides. Chill, covered with plastic wrap, 1 to 3 hours. Bake at 450°F for 10 to 14 minutes, or until biscuits are golden. Makes about 20 biscuits.

NOTE: For drop biscuits, increase milk to ½ cup plus 1½ tablespoons and omit the kneading. Drop rounded tablespoons of dough onto baking sheet about ¾ inch apart and bake as directed.

Each biscuit contains about:
60 calories

50 mg sodium
3 g fat
0 mg cholesterol
Exchanges: 1 bread

CRESCENT ROLLS

    1 envelope active dry yeast
    ¼ cup warm water (105° to 115°F)
    1 cup nonfat milk, heated slightly (about 115°F)
    6 tablespoons egg substitute, or 2 eggs
    ¾ cup plus 2 tablespoons low-calorie
        margarine, softened
  1½ tablespoons fructose
    About 4¼ cups unbleached flour
    ½ teaspoon vegetable oil
    2 additional tablespoons nonfat milk

In a large mixing bowl, dissolve yeast in warm water. Let stand 10 minutes. Mix in heated milk, 3 tablespoons of the egg substitute or 1 egg, 2 tablespoons of the margarine, and fructose. Add 2 cups of the flour and beat with an electric mixer at medium speed for 2 minutes, scraping sides of bowl occasionally. (Or beat by hand until well incorporated.) Stir in 1½ cups of the remaining flour, or enough to make a soft dough. Turn dough out onto a well-floured surface and knead about 5 minutes, adding remaining flour as needed, or until dough is smooth and elastic. Form dough into a ball and place in a bowl lightly greased with the oil. Turn dough ball to grease top side and cover bowl with a towel. Let rise in a warm place until doubled in bulk, about 2 hours.

Roll out dough on a lightly floured surface into an 18-by-12-inch rectangle. Beginning at a long side, spread 4 tablespoons of the margarine over two-thirds of the dough. Fold greased third of dough over center third. Fold ungreased third on top. Rotate dough a quarter turn. Repeat complete procedure two more times (starting with rolling out dough into an 18-by-12-inch rectangle), using remaining margarine. (The dough will look stringy and watery, the layers will separate, and the water content of the margarine will be released, but keep rolling firmly.) Wrap dough in aluminum foil and refrigerate several hours or overnight.

To shape rolls, divide dough into five equal portions. Working with one piece at a time and keeping other portions refrigerated, roll out each portion into a circle about 9 inches in diameter and about ¼ inch thick on a lightly floured board. Cut circle into 8 wedges and roll up each wedge from the wide to the tip end. Form the rolls into crescent shapes and place on ungreased baking sheets, tip side down. When all rolls have been shaped, let rise in a warm place until doubled in bulk, about 45 minutes to 1 hour. Combine remaining 3 tablespoons egg substitute or 1 egg and 2 tablespoons milk and brush mixture on rolls. Bake at 400°F for about 20 minutes or until golden brown. Remove rolls from pans with spatula. Makes about 50 rolls.

Each roll contains approximately:
55 calories
36 mg sodium
2 g fat
0 mg cholesterol
Exchanges: 1 bread

CORN BREAD

2 cups sifted unbleached flour
2 cups yellow cornmeal
¼ cup fructose
2 tablespoons low-sodium baking powder
½ cup low-calorie margarine
1 cup plus 2 tablespoons egg substitute, or 6 eggs
1½ cups nonfat milk

In a mixing bowl, combine flour, cornmeal, fructose, and baking powder and mix well. With a pastry blender, cut margarine into dry ingredients until mixture resembles coarse crumbs. In a small bowl, beat egg substitute or eggs with milk. Add to dry ingredients and stir with a fork until just blended. Pour into a greased 13-by-9-inch baking pan. Bake at 400°F for 25 minutes. Makes 24 servings.

Each 2-by-2-inch slice Corn Bread contains about:
112 calories
49 mg sodium
5 g fat
trace cholesterol
Exchanges: 1 bread, 1 fat

GARLIC BREAD

2 tablespoons low-calorie margarine
1 clove garlic, pressed
1 teaspoon fresh lemon juice
6 slices French Bread (p. 49), toasted on 1 side
Paprika
1 tablespoon grated Romano cheese (optional)
1 tablespoon chopped parsley

Melt margarine in a saucepan and add garlic and lemon juice. Spread garlic-margarine mixture on untoasted side of each bread slice. Sprinkle with paprika and cheese. Place bread slices, buttered side up, on a broiler rack and broil 3 inches from source of heat about 3 minutes or until golden. Sprinkle with parsley. Makes 6 servings.

Each slice Garlic Bread with cheese contains about:
83 calories
58 mg sodium
2 g fat
2 mg cholesterol
Exchanges: 1 bread, 1 fat

FRENCH BREAD

½ cup nonfat milk
1 cup boiling water
1 envelope active dry yeast
¼ cup warm water (105° to 115°F)
1½ tablespoons low-calorie margarine
1 tablespoon plus 2 teaspoons fructose
4 cups sifted unbleached flour
2 tablespoons cornmeal
1 egg white, beaten
1 tablespoon cold water

Scald the milk in a saucepan and add boiling water. Cool to luke-warm (about 85°F). Meanwhile, dissolve yeast in warm water. Let stand 10 minutes, then stir in margarine and milk mixture. Combine fructose and flour in a mixing bowl. Make a well in center and add cooled milk-yeast mixture. Stir thoroughly, but do not knead; the dough will be soft. Form into a ball, cover, and let rise in a warm place, or until doubled in bulk.

Punch down dough and divide into 2 portions. Form each portion into a long loaf on a floured board. Dust bottom of loaves with cornmeal. Place loaves on a greased baking sheet or one lined with parchment paper. Make several ¼-inch-deep slits across tops of loaves. Let rise in a warm place until almost doubled in bulk. Place in oven over a pan of simmering water and bake at 400°F for 15 minutes. Reduce heat to 350°F and bake for 30 minutes, or until golden and crisp. About 5 minutes before loaves are done, mix egg white with cold water and brush on loaves, then finish baking. Makes 2 loaves, 16 slices each.

Bread Sticks

Prepare dough as for French Bread in the preceding recipe. After first rising, roll out half the dough into an 18-by-8-inch rectangle ½-inch thick on a lightly floured board. Cut into 9, 8-by-2-inch strips. Roll each strip into a rope. Hold rope up by one end until stretching stops, then cut in half to make 2 ropes. Place on baking sheet. Repeat with other strips and remaining half of dough. Brush ropes with egg-white glaze and sprinkle with caraway, sesame, cumin, or dill seeds. Let rise in a warm place until barely doubled in bulk, about 20 minutes. Bake at 400°F over a pan of simmering water about 15 minutes or until golden and crisp. Makes 32 bread sticks.

Each slice or stick French Bread contains about:
60 calories
7 mg sodium
0 g fat
0 mg cholesterol
Exchanges: 1 bread

NOTE: To make bread cubes, dice baked French Bread into ½-inch cubes. To toast, bake at 350°F about 7 minutes, or until golden. To make dry bread crumbs, dry bread in 350°F oven 5 minutes or use stale bread. Grind in blender, food processor, or crumble by hand. To make soft bread crumbs, crumble French Bread by hand.

HOLIDAY BREAD

For a decorative touch, sprinkle this bread with an assortment of chopped nuts, orange peel, red apples, or currants before baking, then bake as directed.

¼ cup low-calorie margarine
¼ cup fructose
3 tablespoons egg substitute, or 1 egg
2 tablespoons bourbon or 1 teaspoon rum extract
2 teaspoons vanilla extract
1½ cups unbleached flour
1 teaspoon low-sodium baking powder
1 teaspoon baking soda
½ teaspoon ground cinnamon
¼ teaspoon pumpkin pie spice
½ cup pecans, coarsely chopped
½ cup currants
2 small unpeeled apples, grated
1½ teaspoons grated orange peel

In a mixing bowl, cream together margarine and fructose. Add egg substitute or egg, bourbon, and vanilla extract and beat well. (Mixture will look curdled.) Sift together 1¼ cups of the flour, the baking powder, baking soda, cinnamon, and pie spice. Blend into creamed mixture just until smooth; do not overbeat. Dredge nuts and currants in remaining ¼ cup flour. Fold nut mixture, apples, and orange peel into batter. Spread into an oiled and floured 8-by-3-by-3-inch loaf pan. Bake at 325°F for about 30 minutes, or until a wood pick comes out clean. Cool on wire rack 10 minutes and remove from pan. Cool, then refrigerate. Cut into 24 slices to serve. Keeps about 3 to 4 days. Makes 1 loaf.

NOTE: to decorate top of loaf, reserve 1 tablespoon each of nuts, currants and orange peel. Brush baked loaf with egg white and sprinkle with nuts and fruit. Bake 5 minutes longer or until set.

Each slice contains about:
  64 calories
  63 mg sodium
  3 g fat
  0 mg cholesterol
  Exchanges: 1 bread

POPOVERS

 4 eggs
1¾ cups nonfat milk
 6 tablespoons low-calorie margarine
 2 cups unbleached flour

Beat eggs until frothy. Beat in milk until well blended. Work 5 tablespoons of the margarine into flour gradually. Add flour mixture to milk mixture and beat with electric mixer just until blended. Grease custard cups with remaining 1 tablespoon margarine and fill each with ¼ cup batter. Place on baking sheet and bake at 400°F for 1 hour, or until well browned. Popovers are done when side walls are firm. Let cool, then remove from cups by loosening sides with a sharp knife. Makes 16 popovers.

NOTE: Because the success of this recipe depends on eggs, egg substitute cannot be used. Those on a low-cholesterol diet should notice the cholesterol content.

Each popover contains about:
  89 calories
  69 mg sodium

4 g fat
60 mg cholesterol
Exchanges: 1 bread, 1 fat

RAMONA'S WHOLE WHEAT BREAD

This outstanding low-sodium, low-calorie wheat bread developed by Ramona Ponce, a hospital chef, is so rich that adding a smidgen of butter or anything else to it would be like gilding a lily.

  2 envelopes active dry yeast
1½ cups warm water (105° to 115°F)
  ¾ cup nonfat milk
2½ tablespoons fructose
  5 tablespoons low-calorie margarine
  ⅓ cup low-calorie maple syrup
3½ cups whole wheat flour
3½ cups unbleached flour, sifted
  1 tablespoon poppy seeds or wheat germ

Dissolve yeast in warm water in a large mixing bowl. Let stand 10 minutes. Combine milk, fructose, and margarine in a saucepan and heat, stirring, until fructose dissolves and margarine melts. Blend in maple syrup. Stir warm milk mixture into yeast mixture until smooth. Add 1 cup whole wheat flour and 1 cup unbleached flour to yeast mixture and stir until smooth. Stir remaining whole wheat and unbleached flour into batter and knead 10 minutes, or until smooth and elastic. Form dough into a ball and place in a lightly greased bowl. Turn dough ball to grease top side and cover bowl with plastic wrap. Let rise in a warm place until doubled in bulk, about 1½ hours.

Punch dough down and divide into 2 portions. Form each into a loaf and place in greased 8-by-5-by-3-inch loaf pans. Brush lightly with water and sprinkle with poppy seeds. Let rise in a warm place about 1½ hours, or until almost doubled in bulk. Bake at 400°F for 20 to 25 minutes. Cool on wire racks. Makes 2 loaves, or 25 slices each.

Ramona's Rolls

Prepare dough as for Ramona's Whole Wheat Bread. After first rising, shape the dough into balls to fill 48 greased muffin tin wells about a third full. Let rise until doubled in bulk, about 45 minutes. Brush with water and sprinkle with poppy seeds. Bake at 400°F for 15 to 18 minutes. Makes 48 rolls.

Each slice or roll contains about:
   70 calories
   13 mg sodium
   trace fat
   0 mg cholesterol
   Exchanges: 1 bread

Eggs

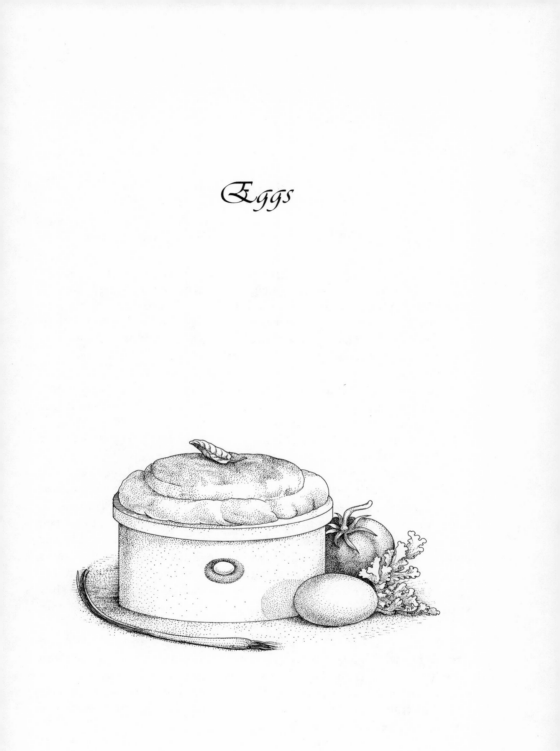

You may wonder what eggs are doing in a book like this. Eggs are nature's wonder food, one of the most nutrient-dense foods in man's diet. They are a source of high-quality protein (7 grams per egg), vitamin B_{12}, and important minerals such as biotin, phosphorus, magnesium, zinc, and copper, among others. Egg yolks are rich in vitamin E and pantothenic acid. So if there is no medical reason to restrict them, eat eggs in moderation. They are one of the least expensive sources of high-quality protein, easy to digest, and easy to prepare, as you will see.

You'll get as much protein from two eggs as two frankfurters, two 2-ounce servings of beef, chicken, or fish, a small meat patty or lamb chop, ½ cup cottage cheese, 2 cups milk, or six pork sausage links. Two eggs are considered one serving.

If you wish to lower the calories, fat, or cholesterol in eggs, use only the white (the protein portion of the egg). Use one egg white for each whole egg called for in recipes. (The yolk houses the cholesterol, fat, and a major portion of the calories.) We have given the recipe for an egg substitute using egg whites. Egg substitute may also be purchased commercially. You'll get the texture, which, in some cases, beats the real thing, if you use the commercial type. You'll also get the lower calories and no cholesterol. However, let's not fool ourselves into thinking that commercial egg substitute is a nutrient replacement for eggs, because it is not. You have only to read the label on the egg substitute package to know that. Our home recipe for egg substitute using only the whites will give you protein without the fat, and no cholesterol, salt, or preservatives, but the texture and flavor of the product to which it is incorporated may suffer a bit. The commercial type, you'll find, is also higher in sodium than the home version. So if you are on a sodium-restricted diet, beware! If using our recipe version, subtract 31 mg sodium and 3 g fat for each 3 tablespoons egg substitute used in the recipe.

56

All the recipes give both egg substitute and eggs optionally to allow for the broadest opportunity to lower calories, fat, and cholesterol or not. The nutrient analysis is given only for the substitute. (We used the nutrient analysis for the commercial product "Second Nature" for convenience.) The reader may refer to the Nutrient Counter (p. 266) to calculate the calories and other nutrients in eggs.

Omelets

FRITTATA

Leave out the cheese if you're in a sodium pinch.

6 zucchini (about 1½ pounds)
2 green onions, sliced
Water or low-sodium Chicken Stock, (p. 40)
¾ cup egg substitute, or 4 eggs
2 cups low-fat cottage cheese
3 tablespoons grated Romano cheese (optional)
⅛ teaspoon pepper
1 tablespoon plus 1 teaspoon vegetable oil

Cook zucchini and green onions in a small amount of water or stock in a covered pan until vegetables are tender, about 5 minutes. Drain well in a colander and dice. Add egg substitute or eggs, cottage cheese, Romano cheese, if desired, and pepper and blend well. Place oil in a 12-by-7-inch or 9-by-9-inch baking pan and heat on stove top until hot. Remove from heat. Pour zucchini-cheese mixture into baking pan and bake at 350°F for 45 to 50 minutes, or until set. Place frittata under broiler a few seconds to brown lightly. Pour off any excess oil. Cut into squares to serve. Makes 16 servings.

Each serving with Romano cheese contains about:
48 calories
143 mg sodium
3 g fat
3 mg cholesterol
Exchanges: 1 vegetable, ¼ meat

HERB OMELET

Endless variations are possible using this omelet as a base. A nourishing, easy to prepare, and economical main dish.

    6 tablespoons egg substitute, or 2 eggs
    1 teaspoon minced parsley
    ¼ teaspoon *each* **dried thyme and tarragon**
    2 teaspoons chopped shallots
    ⅛ teaspoon white pepper
    1 teaspoon low-calorie margarine
    Filling of your choice

Combine egg substitute or eggs, parsley, thyme, tarragon, shallots, and pepper in a bowl and beat until well blended. Melt margarine in a nonstick 7- or 8-inch omelet pan or skillet. Pour egg mixture into the pan and cook over medium heat, lifting the edges as they set so the uncooked portions flow underneath to cook. Continue to cook until the center is dry and set. Top omelet with 2 tablespoons filling of your choice and fold in half. Slide onto serving plate. Makes 1 serving.

    Each omelet without filling contains about:
    95 calories
    176 mg sodium
    12 g fat
    0 mg cholesterol
    Exchanges: 2 meat

Cheese Omelet

Prepare omelet as for Herb Omelet. Fill with 2 tablespoons shredded low-sodium Cheddar or Gouda cheese, or low-fat ricotta or cottage cheese. See Nutrient Analysis for Herb Omelet.

2 tablespoons cheese contains about:

Ricotta or Cottage Cheese	Low-Sodium Cheddar or Gouda
32 calories	110 calories
24 mg sodium	10 mg sodium
1 g fat	9 g fat
10 mg cholesterol	Cholesterol figures not available
Exchanges: ¼ milk	Exchanges: ¼ milk

Florentine Omelet

Prepare omelet as for Herb Omelet, omitting herbs and shallots. Fill with 2 tablespoons Creamed Spinach (p. 142). See Nutrient Analysis for Herb Omelet and Creamed Spinach.

Oriental Omelet

Prepare omelet as for Herb Omelet, omitting herbs and shallots. Fill with 2 tablespoons Chinese Stir-Fry Vegetables (p. 141). See Nutrient Analysis for Herb Omelet and Chinese Stir-Fry Vegetables.

Spanish Omelet

Prepare omelet as for Herb Omelet, omitting herbs and shallots. Fill with 2 tablespoons Spanish Sauce (p. 194). See Nutrient Analysis for Herb Omelet and Spanish Sauce.

OMELET SUPREME

1 teaspoon low-calorie margarine
3 mushrooms, thinly sliced
3 green onions, chopped
2 slices tomato, chopped
¼ teaspoon dried basil
Pinch pepper
6 tablespoons egg substitute, or 2 eggs, beaten
1 tablespoon ricotta cheese (made from partially
   skimmed milk)
1 teaspoon dry white wine

Melt margarine in a nonstick 7- or 8-inch omelet pan or skillet. Add mushrooms, green onions, and tomato and sauté until tender. Remove vegetables from pan and set aside. Combine basil, pepper, and egg substitute or eggs and pour into pan. Cook over medium heat, lifting the edges as they set so the uncooked portions flow underneath to cook. Continue to cook until the center is almost dry and set. Top with mushroom mixture and then ricotta cheese. Sprinkle the filling with wine and fold omelet in half. Slide onto serving plate. Makes 1 serving.

Each omelet contains about:
131 calories
188 mg sodium
12 g fat
5 mg cholesterol
Exchanges: 2 meat, ¼ vegetable

Soufflés *

MUSHROOM SOUFFLE

3 tablespoons low-calorie margarine
1 shallot or small onion, chopped
1½ pounds mushrooms, finely chopped
1½ tablespoons arrowroot
1¼ cups nonfat milk
Pinch cayenne pepper
Pinch ground nutmeg
¾ cup egg substitute, or 4 egg yolks
5 egg whites
1 teaspoon white vinegar

Melt 1 tablespoon of the margarine in a saucepan. Add shallot and mushrooms and cook over medium heat until mushrooms are tender. Remove mushrooms from pan, drain and set aside. Melt remaining 2 tablespoons margarine in the same saucepan. Add arrowroot and cook until smooth. Gradually add milk and cook, stirring, until thickened and smooth, about 5 minutes. Stir in cayenne and nutmeg. Add mushroom mixture to milk mixture and bring to a boil. Remove from heat and stir in egg substitute, a little at a time, or

---

*See dessert chapter for sweet soufflés.

egg yolks, one at a time, until well blended. Let cool slightly. Beat egg whites with vinegar until stiff. Stir about one quarter of the egg whites into the milk mixture to lighten it, then gently fold in remaining whites. Turn into a greased 1-quart soufflé dish and bake at 375°F for 30 minutes, or until golden and puffy. Serve at once. Makes 8 servings.

Each ½ cup serving contains about:
74 calories
148 mg sodium
7 g fat
1 mg cholesterol
Exchanges: 1 meat

SPINACH SOUFFLE

3 tablespoons low-calorie margarine
1 tablespoon chopped shallots or green onion
1 cup chopped fresh spinach, or
    ½ (10-ounce) package frozen chopped spinach,
    thawed, drained, and squeezed dry
1½ tablespoons arrowroot
1¼ cups nonfat milk, heated
Dash *each* cayenne pepper and ground nutmeg
¾ cup plus 3 tablespoons egg substitute, or
    5 eggs, beaten
5 egg whites
1 teaspoon white vinegar

Melt 1 tablespoon of the margarine in a saucepan. Add shallots and sauté until golden. Add spinach and cook until moisture from spinach evaporates. (If using frozen spinach, measure 1 cup and add to pan. Reserve remainder for another use.) Set spinach mixture aside. Melt remaining 2 tablespoons margarine in a separate saucepan. Add arrowroot and stir until smooth. Gradually add hot milk and cook, stirring, until smooth and thickened. Stir in cayenne and nutmeg and bring to a boil. Remove from heat and stir in egg substitute or eggs, a little at a time, until well blended. Add spinach mixture to sauce. Let cool slightly. Beat egg whites with vinegar until stiff. Stir about one-quarter of the egg whites into the milk mixture to lighten it, then gently fold in remaining whites. Turn into a greased 1-quart soufflé dish and bake at 375°F for 30 minutes, or until golden and puffy. Serve at once. Makes 8 servings.

Each ½ cup serving contains about:
    75 calories
    164 mg sodium
    7 g fat
    1 mg cholesterol
    Exchanges: 1 meat, 1 vegetable

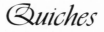

CALIFORNIA QUICHE

    1 medium sweet white onion, halved and
        thinly sliced
    2 teaspoons low-calorie margarine
    ½ pound mushrooms, sliced
    1 teaspoon fresh lemon juice
  1½ teaspoons flour
    ½ cup egg substitute, or 3 eggs
    1 cup evaporated nonfat milk
    Dash ground nutmeg
    Pepper to taste
    1 cup shredded low-sodium Gouda or
        Cheddar cheese
    Quiche Crust (following recipe)
    2 tablespoons grated Romano cheese (optional)
    Dash paprika

Melt margarine in a skillet and sauté onion until tender. Add mushrooms and cook over medium heat until tender, about 3 minutes. Stir in lemon juice, cover, and simmer 2 minutes. Sprinkle with flour and cook, stirring constantly, until mushroom liquid has thickened. Set aside.

Beat egg substitute or eggs lightly and add milk, nutmeg, pepper, and cheese, blending well. Spread mushroom mixture in Quiche Crust and pour in egg mixture. Sprinkle with Romano cheese (without touching pastry) if desired, and paprika. Bake at 350°F for 35 to 40 minutes, or until custard is set and knife inserted near center comes out clean. Cool about 10 minutes before serving. Makes 10 entrée servings.

NOTE: To reheat, place in 350°F oven for 10 to 15 minutes.

Quiche Crust

¾ cup unbleached flour
3 tablespoons vegetable oil
1½ tablespoons nonfat milk
1 egg white, lightly beaten

Place flour in a mixing bowl. Combine oil and milk and add to flour all at once. Mix quickly with a fork until mixture forms into a ball. Roll dough out between sheets of wax paper to a 12-inch circle Line an 8- or 9-inch pie plate with the pastry and crimp edges. Pierce dough in several places with fork. Bake at 450°F for 10 minutes or until golden. Cool before filling.

Each entrée serving contains about:
197 calories
47 mg sodium
12 g fat
1 mg cholesterol
Exchanges: 1 meat, 1 vegetable

ZUCCHINI QUICHE

Sauté 2½ cups sliced zucchini and 1 onion, thinly sliced, in 1 tablespoon vegetable oil until crisp tender. Sprinkle with 1 teaspoon fresh lemon juice. Drain well, then place in Quiche Crust. Prepare egg-milk mixture as directed in California Quiche, substituting ½ teaspoon Herb Blend (p. 206) for the nutmeg. Pour over zucchini mixture and proceed according to directions for California Quiche. Makes 10 entrée servings.

Each entrée serving contains about:
203 calories
47 mg sodium
15 g fat
1 mg cholesterol
Exchanges: 1 meat, 1 vegetable

Crêpes

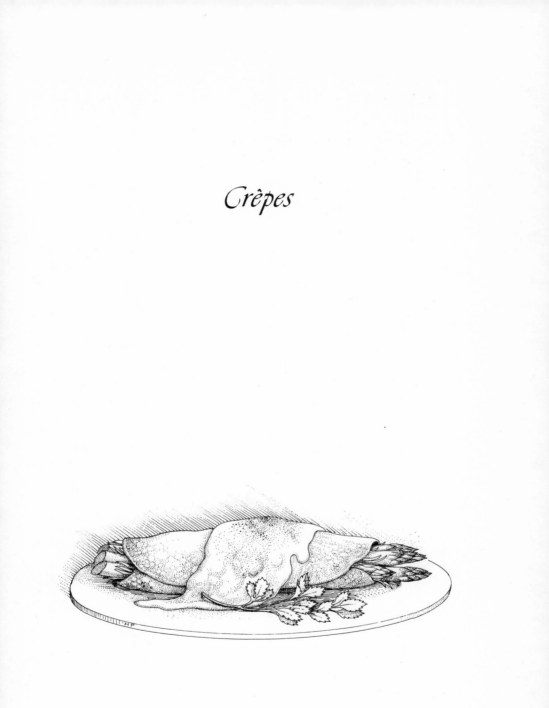

Crêpes are so quick and easy to make, so elegant and glamorous, so versatile in their calorie-cholesterol- salt- and fat-lowering talents, we thought we would devote an entire chapter to them.

There are about 39 calories in each crêpe. That's almost half the calories of bread. Sauces in the filling will increase calories but there's help from a few fat-and-calorie-lowering tricks, such as using nonfat milk for whole milk and replacing flour with arrowroot. Egg substitute (our recipe or store-bought) will cut calories, fat, and cholesterol, too.

We give several of our favorite crêpe and filling recipes. You may come up with filling mixtures of your own. You also can prepare crêpes ahead, stack them between sheets of wax paper, and refrigerate or freeze them to use for impromptu meals. Use the refrigerated crêpes within a week, however. Frozen ones store well up to three months.

If you've never made crêpes before, this is your chance to start. The crêpes should be cooked only on one side, so there is no need to flip and flop like the pros!

Filled Crêpes

CREPES DIVAN

Mornay Sauce (p. 191)
1 teaspoon Worcestershire sauce
½ pound fresh asparagus, cooked and chopped, or
    1 (10-ounce) package frozen cut asparagus, cooked
2 cups shredded cooked turkey meat
6 Feather Crêpes (p. 69)
Dash ground nutmeg

In a mixing bowl, combine half of the Mornay Sauce, the Worcestershire sauce, asparagus, and turkey and mix well. Spoon ¼ cup of mixture in a strip down the center of the unbrowned side of each crêpe. Fold the sides over the filling so they overlap and place seam side down, in a shallow nonstick baking dish in a single layer. Pour remaining Mornay Sauce over crêpes. Sprinkle with nutmeg and bake at 325°F for 20 minutes. Makes 6 servings.

Each serving contains about:
156 calories
136 mg sodium
11 g fat
36 mg cholesterol
Exchanges: 2 meat, ½ bread

CREPES FLORENTINE

1¼ cups Creamed Spinach (p. 142)
6 Feather Crêpes (p. 69)
½ cup Béchamel Sauce (p. 187)
1 tablespoon grated Parmesan cheese

Spoon about 3 tablespoons of the Creamed Spinach in a strip down the center of the unbrowned side of each crêpe. Fold the sides over the filling so they overlap and place seam side down in a shallow nonstick baking pan in a single layer. Spoon Béchamel Sauce over crêpes and sprinkle with cheese. Bake at 350°F for 8 minutes, or until heated through. Place under a broiler for 30 seconds to brown tops. Makes 6 servings.

Each serving contains about:
95 calories
96 mg sodium
1 g fat
1 mg cholesterol
Exchanges: 1 bread, 1 vegetable

CREPES ST. JACQUES

1 pound raw scallops, cooked Alaskan king crab
    meat, or cooked and cleaned shrimp
Water
Mornay Sauce (p. 191)
6 Feather Crêpes (p. 69)
2 tablespoons evaporated nonfat milk
1 tablespoon toasted slivered almonds*

Place scallops in skillet with 1-inch water. Bring to boil, reduce heat, and simmer, covered, 2 minutes. Drain and halve scallops. (If using cooked crab meat or shrimp omit this step.) Stir scallops into one-half of the Mornay Sauce. Spoon about ¼ cup of the filling in a strip down the center of the unbrowned side of each crêpe. Fold the sides over the filling so they overlap and place seam-side down in a shallow nonstick baking dish in a single layer. Stir milk into remaining sauce and spoon over crêpes. Cover pan with aluminum foil and bake at 375°F for 15 minutes. Uncover and bake 5 to 10 minutes longer, or until sauce bubbles. Remove from oven and sprinkle with almonds. Makes 6 servings.

NOTE: Although shrimp is low in calories and fat, it is high in cholesterol. If you are on a cholesterol-restricted diet, use scallops or crab meat.

*To toast almonds, place in a skillet over medium heat and cook, stirring frequently, until golden.

Each serving contains about:
136 calories
242 mg sodium
3 g fat
37 mg cholesterol
Exchanges: 2 meat, ½ bread

RATATOUILLE CREPES

2 cups Ratatouille (p. 146)
8 Feather Crêpes (below)
½ cup low-fat plain yogurt (optional)

Spoon ¼ cup Ratatouille in a strip down the center of the un-browned side of each crêpe. Fold the sides over the filling so they overlap and place seam-side down in a shallow nonstick baking dish in a single layer. Cover pan with aluminum foil and bake at 375°F for 20 minutes, or until heated through. Top each crêpe with 1 table-spoon yogurt, if desired. Makes 8 servings.

Each serving without yogurt contains about:
47 calories
13 mg sodium
1 g fat
0 mg cholesterol
Exchanges: ½ bread, 1 vegetable

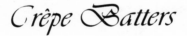

Crêpe Batters

FEATHER CREPES

1 cup unbleached flour
1½ cups nonfat milk
3 tablespoons egg substitute, or 1 egg, beaten
2 teaspoons vegetable oil

In a mixing bowl, combine flour, milk, and egg substitute or egg. Beat with a rotary beater or wire whisk until blended. Chill batter. Lightly grease a 6-inch nonstick skillet or crêpe pan with some of the oil and place over medium heat until pan is hot. Remove pan from heat and spoon in about 2 tablespoons of the batter. Lift and tilt the skillet to spread the batter evenly over the pan bottom. Return pan to medium heat and cook crêpe until lightly browned on underside. Turn crêpe out onto paper toweling. (Crêpe will slide easily from pan when done.) Repeat until all crêpes are cooked, greasing skillet as necessary. Makes about 18 crêpes.

Each crêpe contains about:
36 calories
13 mg sodium
1 g fat
trace cholesterol
Exchanges: ½ bread

Feather Wheat Crêpes

Proceed as directed for Feather Crêpes, substituting 1¼ cups whole wheat flour for the unbleached flour, increasing nonfat milk to 1¾ cups, and substituting low-calorie margarine for the vegetable oil. Makes about 18 crêpes.

Each crêpe contains about:
39 calories
14 mg sodium
1 g fat
trace cholesterol
Exchanges: ½ bread

FEATHER CREPE CUPS

1 cup all-purpose flour
1½ cups nonfat milk
½ teaspoon fructose
3 tablespoons egg substitute, or 1 egg
3 tablespoons low-calorie margarine

In a mixing bowl, combine flour, milk, fructose, and egg substitute or egg. Beat until blended. Melt ⅛ teaspoon of the margarine in a 6-inch nonstick skillet or crêpe pan placed over medium heat. Remove from heat and spoon in about 1 tablespoon of batter. Lift and tilt skillet to spread batter evenly into a 5-inch circle. Return pan to heat. Brown crêpe on one side only and slip onto paper toweling. (Crêpe will slide easily from pan when done.) Continue until all crêpes are cooked, using ⅛ teaspoon margarine for cooking each crêpe.

Invert 18 custard cups on baking sheets. Grease outside of cups with remaining margarine. (You may need to make the crêpe cups in batches, depending on the number of custard cups you have.) Place a crêpe, browned side up, onto each custard cup. Press crêpe lightly to fit cup. Bake at 375°F until crisp, about 20 to 25 minutes. Use a knife tip to remove crêpes from cups. Cool and stack, wrapped in plastic wrap, until ready to use. Makes 18.

Each crêpe cup contains about:
40 calories
32 mg sodium
1 g fat
0 mg cholesterol
Exchanges: ½ bread

Fish and Shellfish

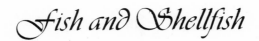

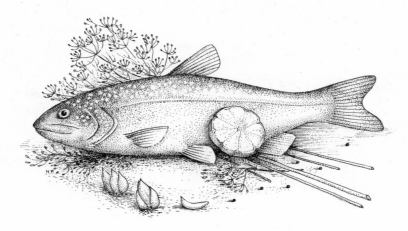

$\mathcal{F}$ish is a *Light Style* natural. It's low in calories (about 100 per 4 ounces for most fish), higher in poly-unsaturated fats, and relatively lower in cholesterol than beef.

Most lean fish is generally classified as white flesh fish, with less than 5 percent fat. But even the so-called fatty fish, such as mackerel and salmon, contain only 5 to 15 percent fat, and that's 20 percent less than most red meat.

Fish is especially high in B vitamins and provides important minerals, such as potassium, phosphorus, iron, iodine, fluoride and zinc. A 4-ounce serving of fish, in fact, provides one-third of the recommended daily adult protein allowance, making it a fine protein choice several times a week.

You'll reduce calories, cholesterol, and fat, however, if you poach, rather than fry, fish. Sautéing is fine if you use minimum amounts of fat and/or a nonstick cooking utensil. Most any cooking method lends itself to an infinite variety of preparations. Poached fish can be served with most any sauce, as can cold fish with cold sauces.

Fresh herbs and vegetables enhance the flavor of fish cooked without salt, especially when baking and broiling fish.

Seafood is high in protein and low in fat and calories. Some shellfish is also very high in cholesterol, so it's best to check the nutrient analysis for each recipe or the Nutrient Counter (p. 266) for the cholesterol content of a specific shellfish if you are watching cholesterol for medical reasons. All shellfish except shrimp, however, are now on the American Heart Association's "okay" list for people on cholesterol diets.

We've included several recipes for scallops because they're lower in fat than any other shellfish. If sodium is your worry, however, avoid scallops and shrimp and stick to whitefish or other fresh-water fish.

74

A reminder about cooking fish properly. Fish has naturally tender flesh and requires a short cooking time. Overcooking toughens protein and creates a rubbery texture. Fragile fish also needs a light touch when handling. Transfer fish with two spatulas to prevent breaking. You'll also improve the chances of top-quality texture, flavor, and vitamin content if you use fresh fish. It's worth a trip to the fish market for the extra quality.

Fish

CLASSIC SOLE

2 tablespoons low-calorie margarine
3 or 4 shallots, finely minced
½ pound mushrooms, sliced
⅓ cup dry white wine
Juice of 1 lemon
6 (4-ounce) fish fillets, such as sole, haddock,
    halibut, or snapper (about 1½ pounds)
¾ cup Sauce Velouté (p. 197)
6 asparagus spears, cooked and kept warm (p. 138)

Heat margarine in a large skillet. Add shallots and mushrooms and sauté 2 minutes. Add 2 tablespoons of the wine and sauté 1 minute longer, or until mushrooms are tender. Remove mushroom mixture from skillet; set aside and keep hot.

Add remaining wine, lemon juice, and fillets to skillet and cook until fillets are tender, about 3 minutes on each side. Place fillets on a heated platter and top with Sauce Velouté. Arrange asparagus spears and mushrooms over fish. Makes 6 servings.

Each serving with sauce contains about:
  150 calories
  70 mg sodium
  3 g fat
  70 mg cholesterol
  Exchanges: 3 meat

DILLY TROUT IN A POUCH

6 (4-ounce) lake trout, split and cleaned
White pepper to taste
6 fresh sprigs dill or fennel, or
    1½ teaspoons dill weed
2 shallots, minced
3 tablespoons dry Sherry
½ cup Fish Stock (p. 41)
2 teaspoons low-calorie margarine
6 lemon slices
Lemon wedges

Rub each trout inside and out with pepper. Place a sprig of dill or fennel or some of the dill weed in each cavity. Cut out 6 (6-inch) circles of aluminum foil. Fold each circle in half and pinch the corners to make a "boat" shape. Fit each trout into a foil boat and sprinkle with shallots. Mix together Sherry and stock and pour over each trout. Dot each with bits of margarine and top with a lemon slice. Bring edges of foil up to completely enclose fish and pinch foil together securely. (The shape of the pouch should resemble a turnover.) Place trout pouches in a baking dish and bake at 450°F for 25 minutes or until trout are tender when tested with a fork.

To serve, place pouches on a serving platter, and with scissors cut open tops of pouches so that each diner may lift out the trout easily. Garnish with lemon wedges. Makes 6 servings.

    Each serving contains about:
      243 calories
      27 mg sodium
      13 g fat
      76 mg cholesterol
      Exchanges: 4 meat

MARINE KEBABS

Serve this colorful kebab over a bed of rice for a complete meal.

   ½ pound scallops
   12 cherry tomatoes
   ¼ pound swordfish, cut in 1-inch cubes
   1 green bell pepper, cut in small squares
   1 onion, cut in 6 wedges
   ¼ pound halibut, cut in 1-inch cubes
   2 tablespoons low-calorie margarine
   1 tablespoon fresh lemon juice
   Lemon wedges
   Tartar Sauce (p. 210), optional

Alternately thread scallops, cherry tomatoes, swordfish, green pepper, onion, and halibut on each of 6 metal skewers. Melt margarine in a small saucepan placed over low heat. Add lemon juice and heat through. Brush kebabs with some of the margarine-lemon mixture and place on rack in a broiler pan. Broil 4 inches from source of heat about 4 minutes on each side, basting often. Arrange on serving platter and garnish with lemon wedges. Serve with Tartar Sauce, if desired. Makes 6 servings.

   Each skewer without sauce contains about:
   116 calories
   146 mg sodium
   3 g fat
   53 mg cholesterol
   Exchanges: 3 meat

POACHED SEA BASS

This simple, but elegant, treatment of fish is low in calories.

   Court Bouillon (following recipe)
   6 (4-ounce) sea bass, salmon, haddock, whitefish,
      other fish fillets or steaks (about 1½ pounds)
   1 tablespoon chopped parsley
   Lemon wedges

Place Court Bouillon in a large skillet and heat to a simmer. Place fish in Court Bouillon, cover, and simmer until fish becomes creamy white and flakes easily when tested with a fork, about 12 to 15 minutes. Carefully remove fish to a heated serving platter. Sprinkle with parsley and garnish with lemon wedges. Makes 6 servings.

Each serving contains about:
110 calories
83 mg sodium
3 g fat
68 mg cholesterol
Exchanges: 3 meat

Court Bouillon

¾ cups dry white wine
¾ cups water
½ small onion, sliced
½ stalk celery, cut up
½ carrot, sliced
1 sprig parsley
1 bay leaf

Combine wine, water, onion, celery, carrots, parsley, and bay leaf in a large saucepan. Bring to a boil, reduce heat, and simmer, covered, 15 minutes. Strain through a fine sieve or cheesecloth. Makes 1½ cups.

Each ½ cup contains about:
15 calories
trace sodium
trace fat
trace cholesterol
Exchanges: negligible

SOLE AMANDINE

6 (4-ounce) sole, perch, or haddock fillets
    (about 1½ pounds)
Flour
2 tablespoons plus 1 teaspoon low-calorie margarine
1 teaspoon vegetable oil
Juice of 1 lemon
1 clove garlic, minced
¼ cup slivered almonds, chopped
¼ cup dry white wine
1 tablespoon chopped parsley
White pepper to taste

Dust fish lightly with flour. Heat 2 tablespoons of the margarine and the oil in a skillet. Add fillets and sauté about 2 to 3 minutes on each side, or until fish becomes creamy white and flakes easily when tested with a fork. Remove fish to a heated serving platter and sprinkle with lemon juice.

Melt remaining 1 teaspoon margarine in skillet placed over medium heat. Add garlic, almonds, and wine and cook, stirring briskly for 30 seconds, or until light brown in color. Spoon sauce over fish and sprinkle with parsley and pepper. Makes 6 servings.

NOTE: Whole trout may be used in place of fillets.

Each serving contains about:
  168 calories
  110 mg sodium
  6 g fat
  60 mg cholesterol
  Exchanges: 3 meat

SWORDFISH PIQUANT

3 tablespoons low-calorie margarine
4 large cloves garlic, minced or pressed
Juice of 1 lemon
6 (4-ounce) swordfish steaks, 1 inch thick
    (about 1½ pounds)
2 tablespoons chopped parsley
2 lemons, cut in wedges
Paprika

Melt margarine in a saucepan over low heat. Add garlic and lemon juice and heat briefly to blend flavors. Brush half of the margarine-garlic mixture on one side of each swordfish steak. Place, basted side up, on a broiler pan and broil 4 inches from source of heat about 6 minutes. Turn steaks over, brush with remaining margarine-garlic mixture, and broil 6 minutes on second side, or until fish flakes easily with a fork. Place on a heated platter and garnish with chopped parsley, lemon wedges, and paprika. Makes 6 servings.

Each serving contains about:
    159 calories
    96 mg sodium
    9 g fat
    57 mg cholesterol
    Exchanges: 4 meat

SOLE VERONIQUE

A modern variation on a classic theme cuts calories drastically.

   2 shallots or green onions (white part only), minced
   2 tablespoons low-calorie margarine
   6 (4-ounce) fillets of sole (about 1½ pounds)
   ½ cup dry white wine
   ¼ cup water
1½ teaspoons arrowroot
   ¼ cup plus 1 teaspoon nonfat milk
   ¼ cup evaporated nonfat milk
   ½ cup small seedless white grapes
   2 tablespoons egg substitute, or
         1 egg yolk, beaten
   White pepper to taste
   2 tablespoons slivered almonds, toasted* (optional)

Sauté shallots in 1 tablespoon of the margarine in skillet until tender. Add fish fillets, wine, and water. Cut a circle of wax paper the size of the skillet, grease one side, and place it grease side down over fish. Bring liquid to a boil, reduce heat, and simmer, covered, until fish is tender when tested with a fork, about 12 to 15 minutes. Carefully transfer fillets to a heated serving platter.

In a small saucepan, melt remaining 1 tablespoon margarine. Mix arrowroot with 1 teaspoon nonfat milk and stir into margarine until smooth. Gradually add ¼ cup *each* nonfat milk and evaporated nonfat milk and bring to a boil. Reduce heat and cook, stirring, until thickened and smooth. Stir ¼ cup of the hot sauce into egg substitute, then return to sauce in pan. Cook and stir until blended. Add grapes and heat through. Season to taste with pepper. Spoon sauce over fish. Sprinkle with toasted slivered almonds, if desired. Makes 6 servings.

* To toast almonds, place in a dry pan over medium heat and heat, stirring, until golden.

   Each serving with almonds contains about:
   154 calories
   158 mg sodium
   3 g fat
   62 mg cholesterol
   Exchanges: 4 meat

Fish and Shellfish   81

CRAB-STUFFED SOLE

2 tablespoons low-calorie margarine
2 tablespoons dry white wine
2 tablespoons fresh lemon juice
6 (4-ounce) fillets of sole (about 1½ pounds)
¾ cup Sauce Velouté (p. 197)
¼ pound shredded Alaskan king crab meat
    (fresh or frozen)
1 tablespoon chopped parsley

Melt margarine in a large skillet. Add wine and lemon juice. Place
sole in skillet and simmer, covered, 3 minutes or until fish becomes
creamy white and flakes easily when tested with a fork. Combine
¼ cup of the Sauce Velouté and the crab meat in a small saucepan
and heat through. Place 1 tablespoon of the crab meat mixture in the
center of each fillet. Roll up jellyroll fashion and secure with wood
picks. Arrange stuffed rolls in a nonstick baking pan. Pour remaining
Sauce Velouté over fish. Bake at 350°F 10 minutes. Sprinkle with
parsley. Makes 6 servings.

    NOTE: Canned crab meat has a very high salt content. We suggest
that those watching their salt intake use only fresh or frozen Alaskan
king crab meat.

    Each serving with sauce contains about:
    136 calories
    125 mg sodium
    4 g fat
    75 mg cholesterol
    Exchanges: 4 meat

WHITEFISH A LA PORT

2 tablespoons honey, or 1 tablespoon fructose
½ cup port wine or dry Sherry
Juice of 2 lemons
1 teaspoon dill weed, or 1 sprig fresh dill, minced
6 (4-ounce) whitefish, snapper, or sea bass fillets
    (about 1½ pounds)
Parsley or dill sprigs
Paprika

Blend together honey, port, lemon juice, and dill in a small bowl. Brush fish with mixture, reserving some for basting. Broil fillets 4 inches from source of heat, basting often with marinade, 3 minutes on each side, or until fish is creamy white and flakes easily when tested with a fork. Garnish with parsley and dust with paprika. Makes 6 servings.

Each serving contains about:
138 calories
76 mg sodium
1 g fat
65 mg cholesterol
Exchanges: 4 low-fat meat

Shellfish

ABALONE MEUNIERE

The classic sauce used in this recipe is quick, tasty, and simple to make. It is also excellent with veal, chicken, or any fish.

2 tablespoons low-calorie margarine
1 clove garlic, minced
½ pound mushrooms, sliced
2 tablespoons dry white wine
1 tablespoon vegetable oil
1 tablespoon flour
Pepper to taste
1 pound abalone, cut into 6 thin steaks
   and pounded
¼ cup nonfat milk
1 tablespoon chopped parsley
2 teaspoons fresh lemon juice
Lemon wedges

Melt 1 tablespoon of the margarine in a skillet. Add garlic and mushrooms and sauté about 2 minutes. Add wine and sauté until mushrooms are tender and liquid is almost absorbed; set aside and keep hot.

In another skillet, heat remaining margarine and oil. Season flour with pepper. Dredge abalone steaks lightly in seasoned flour mixture, then dip in milk. Place in the skillet and cook about 1 minute on each side. Remove to a heated platter. Spoon mushrooms over abalone and sprinkle with parsley and lemon juice. Garnish with lemon wedges. Makes 6 servings.

Each serving contains about:
  149 calories
  42 mg sodium (content unavailable for abalone)
  4 g fat (content unavailable for abalone)
  73 mg cholesterol
  Exchanges: 3 meat

LIME-LACED LOBSTER TAILS

  6 (6-ounce) lobster tails
  ¼ cup low-calorie margarine
  ¼ cup fresh lime or lemon juice
  2 cloves garlic, minced
  ⅛ teaspoon paprika
  ⅛ teaspoon white pepper
  1 teaspoon finely chopped parsley

With scissors, snip off the soft undercovering of each lobster tail. Remove the meat from the shell and clean and reserve shells. Cut meat in small pieces and place in a shallow dish. Melt margarine in a small saucepan. Add lime juice, garlic, paprika, pepper, and parsley. Pour over lobster and marinate in the refrigerator for 1 hour.

Remove meat from marinade, reserving marinade for basting. Stuff meat back into shells. Place shells on a broiler pan and broil 4 inches from source of heat about 10 minutes, basting often with reserved marinade. Makes 6 servings.

NOTE: 6 ounces of lobster includes the shell.

Each serving contains about:
  123 calories

226 mg sodium
4 g fat
72 mg cholesterol
Exchanges: 3 meat

PICNIC LOBSTER

6 (1-pound) live lobsters
Drawn Margarine (p. 189), or
    Seafood Cocktail Sauce (p. 208)
Lemon wedges

Add enough water to a large kettle so the lobsters will be completely immersed when you plunge them. Bring water to a rolling boil. Immerse live lobsters in water head first, and allow the water to return to a boil. Reduce heat and simmer about 20 minutes, or until lobster shells are bright red. Drain. Serve with small bowl of Drawn Margarine or Seafood Cocktail Sauce and lemon wedges. Cut lobsters on underside, separating shell from meat. Use lobster fork or shellfish fork to pick out meat. Makes 6 servings.

Each lobster without sauce contains about:
    104 calories
    238 mg sodium
    3 g fat
    110 mg cholesterol
    Exchanges: 3 meat

SCALLOPS IN CIDER

½ cup Fish Stock (p. 41)
½ cup unsweetened apple cider
 2 teaspoons minced shallots
¼ teaspoon dried tarragon
½ pound mushrooms, thinly sliced
1½ pounds scallops or cleaned shrimp
  Pepper to taste
 1 tablespoon chopped parsley

Combine stock, cider, shallots, tarragon, mushrooms, and scallops in a skillet and sprinkle with pepper. Bring to a boil, reduce heat, and simmer, uncovered, 4 minutes or until scallops are tender. With a slotted spoon, remove scallops and mushrooms to a heated serving platter. Bring pan liquid to a boil and boil 3 to 4 minutes, or until liquid is reduced by one-third. Spoon pan liquid over scallop mixture and sprinkle with parsley. Makes 6 servings.

NOTE: Do not use shrimp if on an extremely low-cholesterol diet.

Each serving contains about:
124 calories
312 mg sodium
trace fat
44 mg cholesterol
Exchanges: 4 meat

SCALLOPS MARCUS

A squeeze of lemon juice over the scallops keeps them creamy white.

2 tablespoons low-calorie margarine
2 tablespoons dry white wine
1 clove garlic, minced
1 sprig parsley, finely chopped
1½ pounds scallops
2 tablespoons fresh lemon juice
Lemon wedges

Melt margarine in a small saucepan. Add wine, garlic, and parsley and blend thoroughly. Sprinkle scallops with lemon juice and place in a baking dish. Pour margarine-wine mixture over scallops and bake at 350°F for 15 minutes. Garnish with lemon wedges. Makes 6 servings.

Each serving contains about:
113 calories
344 mg sodium
2 g fat
44 mg cholesterol
Exchanges: 4 meat

Poultry and Game

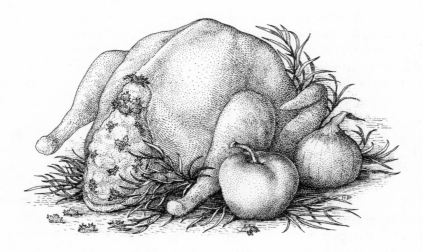

$\mathcal{J}$t's easy to see why chicken is fast becoming America's favorite meat. It's naturally *Light Style* in calories, fats, and cholesterol (if you remove the skin); easy and quick to cook; versatile in its preparation possibilities; and top quality in protein, vitamins, and minerals. Chicken is also lower in cost than most other meats, fish, and even some cheeses.

If you check the Nutrient Counter (p. 266) you will note that game is rather high in calories and fat, and that dark meat tends to be slightly higher in both calories and fat than light.

Our *Light Style* recipes show you how to keep the calories and fat of poultry and game low and flavor high. We emphasize the use of the least fatty poultry cuts, such as the breasts. The skin and any excess fat is removed to reduce calories, fat, and cholesterol further. We use calorie-lowering cooking methods, such as broiling, baking, light sautéing, and barbecuing, and suggest the use of nonstick cooking utensils if possible.

We go light on fats and use polyunsaturated fats whenever possible. Arrowroot and cornstarch replace flour in recipes calling for thickening. Salt is omitted completely and replaced with effective seasonings, herbs, spices, and wines.

Another bonus: All the recipes calling for chicken breasts are interchangeable with veal and turkey cutlets or other meat cutlets for a change of pace in meal planning. You can also substitute one fowl for another in any recipe, but use the thermometer chart on page 293 as a cooking guide.

You will notice a shrinkage factor after cooking. We have compensated for shrinkage in the nutrient analysis of each recipe.

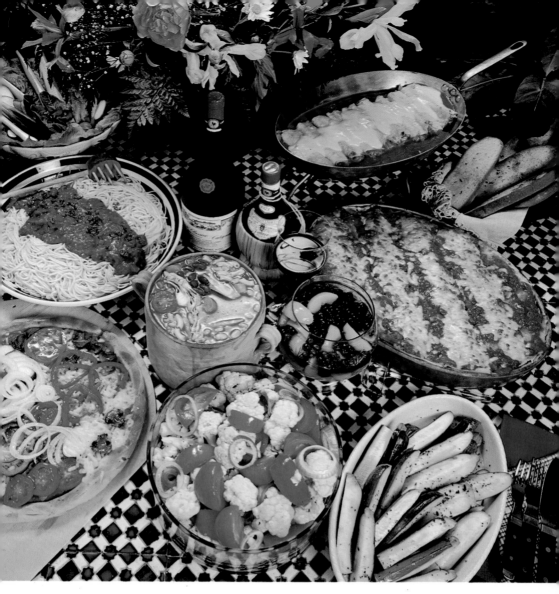

An Italian feast with half the calories and a third the sodium of the regular dishes features, clockwise from lower left: Pizza, a medley of vegetables and low-fat cheese; Spaghetti with Italian Meat Sauce, made with lean beef and fresh tomatoes; Kathy's Cannelloni, using béchamel and tomato sauces, both low in fat and sodium; Garlic Bread, spread with low-calorie margarine; Lasagna made with low-fat ricotta cheese and sauce; steamed Zucchini Oregano; and Tomato Cauliflower Salad, easy on oil. At center is Hearty Minestrone, a salt-free, low-fat, high-taste soup, and Peaches Galliano, a blueberry and peach bowl splashed with Galliano.

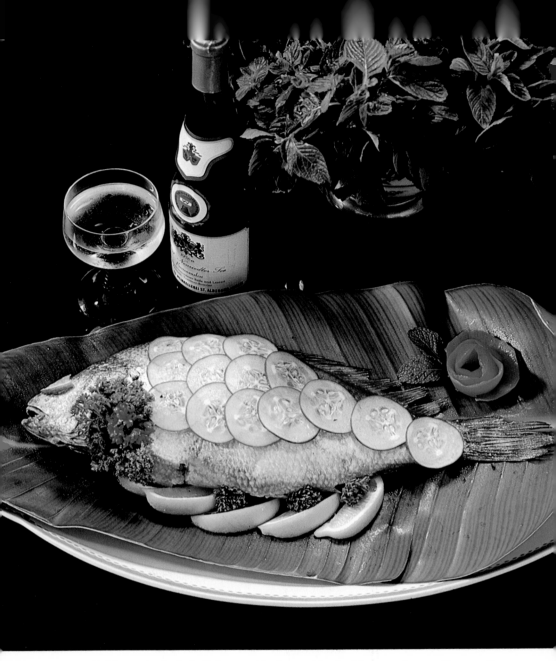

Cold poached whole fish on a ti leaf, garnished with cucumber and lemon slices, a tomato "rose," and sweet william, is ready to serve with a chilled sauce such as Curry Mayonnaise or Mock Hollandaise.

Chicken

BARBECUED CHICKEN

3 whole chicken breasts (about 1½ pounds
    boned weight)
1½ teaspoons Worcestershire sauce*
¼ cup water
½ cup Catsup (p. 203)
¼ cup unsweetened pineapple juice
1 teaspoon brown sugar substitute, or
    1 tablespoon fructose
Pepper to taste
2 tablespoons low-calorie margarine, melted

Skin, bone, and split chicken breasts. Pound into thin cutlets between sheets of wax paper with a mallet. In a saucepan, combine Worcestershire sauce, water, Catsup, pineapple juice, brown sugar substitute, and pepper. Bring to a boil, reduce heat, and simmer 10 minutes. Combine sauce and margarine in a shallow baking dish. Coat chicken cutlets with mixture and marinate for 15 minutes, turning occasionally to coat all sides. Grill over charcoal or broil 3 minutes on each side, or bake at 350°F for 15 minutes. Makes 6 servings.

NOTE: This sauce is also delicious on ground beef patties and pork chops.

*French's Worcestershire sauce is lower in sodium content than other brands, to our knowledge.

Each serving contains about:
    135 calories
    138 mg sodium
    5 g fat
    59 mg cholesterol
    Exchanges: 3 meat

CHICKEN CASHEW

3 whole chicken breasts (about 1½ pounds
    boned weight)
2 tablespoons low-calorie margarine
2 cloves garlic, minced
1 teaspoon minced ginger root
¼ cup unsalted cashews
2 teaspoons fresh lemon juice
½ pound asparagus spears, cooked (p. 138)

Skin, bone, and split chicken breasts. Cut meat into ¼-inch-wide strips. Melt margarine in a large skillet and add garlic, ginger, cashews, lemon juice, and chicken. Cook, tossing gently, until golden, about 5 minutes. Garnish with asparagus spears. Makes 6 servings.

Each serving contains about:
   157 calories
   118 mg sodium
   7 g fat
   59 mg cholesterol
   Exchanges: 3 meat

CHICKEN MARENGO

3 whole chicken breasts (about 1½ pounds
    boned weight)
2 tablespoons low-calorie margarine
1½ cloves garlic, finely minced
2 shallots, finely chopped
2½ cups low-sodium Chicken Stock, (p. 40)
5 medium tomatoes, peeled and chopped
1½ medium onions, cut in wedges
1 pound mushrooms, sliced
1 bay leaf
1 tablespoon Herb Blend (p. 206)
1 tablespoon chopped parsley
¼ cup dry Sherry

Skin, bone, and split chicken breasts. Pound into thin cutlets between sheets of waxed paper with a mallet. Melt margarine in a skillet. Add chicken, garlic, and shallots, and sauté until chicken is golden brown, 3 to 4 minutes on each side. Remove chicken and set aside. Add stock, tomatoes, onions, mushrooms, bay leaf and Herb Blend to skillet. Bring to a boil, reduce heat, and simmer 7 to 10 minutes. Return chicken to skillet, add Sherry, and heat through. Sprinkle with parsley. Makes 6 servings.

Each 3 ounce serving contains about:
159 calories
139 mg sodium
5 g fat
60 mg cholesterol
Exchanges: 3 meat, 1 vegetable

CHICKEN ALLA MARSALA

3 whole chicken breasts (about 1½ pounds boned
    weight), or 1½ pounds veal scallops
¼ cup flour
Pepper to taste
3 tablespoons low-calorie margarine
¼ cup minced shallots
1 clove garlic, minced
½ pound mushrooms, sliced
½ cup sweet Marsala wine

Skin, bone, and split chicken breasts. Pound into thin cutlets be-tween sheets of wax paper with a mallet. (You need only to pound veal scallops.) Mix together flour and pepper and dredge chicken lightly in seasoned flour, shaking off excess. In a skillet, melt 2 table-spoons of the margarine and sauté shallots, garlic, and mushrooms until vegetables are tender. Remove vegetables and set aside. Melt remaining 1 tablespoon margarine in same skillet, add chicken and sauté 2 to 3 minutes on each side, or until golden. Add Marsala and reserved mushroom mixture and cook 1 minute longer or until tender. Remove chicken and mushrooms from skillet with a slotted spoon and arrange on a heated platter. Bring liquid remaining in pan to a brisk boil and cook until reduced to a thin syrupy glaze. Pour glaze over chicken and mushrooms. Makes 6 servings.

Each serving contains about:
186 calories
138 mg sodium
6 g fat
59 mg cholesterol
Exchanges: 3 meat

ENCHILADAS SUIZA

2 whole chicken breasts, boned and skinned
   (1 pound boned weight)
1 cup low-sodium Chicken Stock (p. 40)
6 corn tortillas
Suiza Sauce (following recipe)
2 tablespoons low-calorie sour cream
Chopped green onions

Place chicken breasts in skillet and add chicken stock. Bring to a boil, reduce heat, cover, and simmer 10 to 15 minutes, or until chicken breasts are tender. Remove chicken breasts from stock, cool and shred meat. Set aside.

Heat tortillas on ungreased griddle until piping hot and softened. Dip tortilla in Suiza Sauce. Place about 2 tablespoons shredded chicken in center of each tortilla and fold over once. Place on serving platter. Repeat with remaining tortillas and filling. Pour remaining Suiza Sauce over enchiladas. Garnish each enchilada with 1 teaspoon sour cream and sprinkle with green onions. Makes 6 servings.

Suiza Sauce

4 tomatoes, peeled, or 1 (1-pound) can
   low-sodium tomatoes, drained
1 large onion, chopped
1 tablespoon corn oil
1 cup evaporated nonfat milk

Combine tomatoes and onion in a blender container and blend until smooth. Heat oil in a skillet and add tomato mixture. Bring to a boil, reduce heat to low, and simmer, uncovered, 30 minutes or until slightly thickened, stirring occasionally. Stir in milk gradually. Heat through.

Each enchilada with sauce contains about:
210 calories
100 mg sodium
3 g fat
42 mg cholesterol
Exchanges: 2 meat, ½ bread, 1 B vegetable

LEMON CHICKEN

3 whole chicken breasts (about 1½ pounds
    boned weight)
2 tablespoons Soy Sauce (p. 209)
2 tablespoons gin, vodka, or other high-proof
    alcoholic beverage
1 tablespoon Chinese-style sesame seed oil
½ teaspoon ginger juice*
2 teaspoons arrowroot or cornstarch
1 tablespoon water
1½ to 2 tablespoons fresh lemon juice
1 teaspoon grated lemon peel
1 teaspoon fructose, or
    sugar substitute to equal 2 teaspoons sugar
¼ cup low-sodium Chicken Stock (p. 40)

Skin, bone, and split chicken breasts. Mix together the Soy Sauce and gin, rub the mixture over the chicken and let it marinate in the refrigerator about 1 hour, turning occasionally. Remove chicken from marinade and dice. Heat oil and ginger juice in a saucepan or wok over moderately low heat. Add chicken and cook, stirring constantly, until golden, about 3 minutes. Remove chicken with a slotted spoon and set aside. Dissolve arrowroot in water and add to pan. Stir until smooth. Stir in lemon juice, lemon peel, fructose, and stock. Cook over low heat, stirring, until thickened. Add reserved chicken and heat through. Makes 6 servings.

* To extract juice from ginger, place a 1-inch piece of ginger root in a garlic press and squeeze. Use more ginger as needed to make ½ teaspoon juice.

Each serving contains about:
146 calories
103 mg sodium
5 g fat
59 mg cholesterol
Exchanges: 3 meat

CHICKEN-MUSHROOM SAUTE

3 whole chicken breasts (about
    1½ pounds boned weight)
2 tablespoons low-calorie margarine
¾ cup dry white wine
2 cloves garlic, minced
1 pound mushrooms, sliced
½ teaspoon paprika
¼ cup flour
2 teaspoons fresh lemon juice
1 tablespoon finely chopped parsley
White pepper to taste
1 teaspoon arrowroot

Skin, bone, and split chicken breasts. Pound into thin cutlets between sheets of wax paper with a mallet; set aside. Heat 1 tablespoon of the margarine in a skillet. Add ½ cup of the wine, garlic, and mushrooms and cook until mushrooms are tender. Remove mushrooms with a slotted spoon and keep hot; reserve liquid in pan.

Mix together paprika and flour and dredge chicken lightly in the mixture. Add remaining 1 tablespoon margarine, lemon juice, parsley, and white pepper to reserved pan liquid, and heat until margarine melts. Add chicken and cook until tender, about 2 to 3 minutes on each side. Remove chicken and mushrooms with a slotted spoon and arrange on a heated serving platter; reserve pan liquid. Dissolve arrowroot in remaining ¼ cup wine and add to pan liquid. Stir over low heat until thickened. Pour sauce over chicken and mushrooms. Makes 6 servings.

Each serving contains about:
  155 calories
  123 mg sodium
  3 g fat
  59 mg cholesterol
  Exchanges: 3 meat, 1 vegetable

CHICKEN ORIENTAL

1 tablespoon safflower oil
2 cloves garlic, minced
3 whole chicken breasts (about 1½ pounds
  boned weight), skinned, boned, and cut
  into 1-inch cubes
2 cups chopped celery
½ pound mushrooms, sliced
½ pound bean sprouts
1 teaspoon minced ginger root or
  ½ teaspoon ground ginger
⅛ teaspoon pepper
½ teaspoon cornstarch
1 tablespoon water
2 tablespoons Soy Sauce (p. 209)
3 cups Steamed Rice (p. 132)

Heat oil in a hot skillet or wok until oil smokes. Add the garlic and stir-fry for 10 seconds. Add the chicken and stir-fry until cooked (about 4 minutes). Add celery, mushrooms, ginger, and pepper and sauté until celery is tender—about 5 minutes—stirring frequently. Dissolve cornstarch in water; then mix in soy sauce. Push aside chicken and vegetables and stir cornstarch mixture into juices. Cook, stirring frequently, until mixture thickens. Divide into 6 equal portions and spoon each serving over ½ cup rice. Makes 6 servings.

Each ½ cup serving with ½ cup rice contains about:
  224 calories
  229 mg sodium
  5 g fat
  60 mg cholesterol
  Exchanges: 3 meat, ½ vegetable, 1 bread

CHICKEN PICCATA

3 whole chicken breasts (about 1½ pounds
    boned weight), or 1½ pounds of veal scallops
¼ cup flour
Pepper to taste
3 tablespoons low-calorie margarine
¾ cup low-sodium Chicken Stock (p. 40)
1½ tablespoons fresh lemon juice
6 paper-thin lemon slices

Skin, bone, and split chicken breasts. Pound into thin cutlets between sheets of wax paper with a mallet. Mix together flour and pepper and dredge chicken lightly in seasoned flour, shaking off excess. Melt 2 tablespoons of the margarine in a skillet and sauté chicken 2 to 3 minutes on each side, or until golden. Remove chicken and set aside. Add ½ cup of the stock and lemon juice to skillet, bring to a boil, and boil 1 to 2 minutes. Return chicken to skillet and place 1 lemon slice on each cutlet. Cover and simmer 7 to 10 minutes, or until chicken is tender. Remove chicken with a slotted spoon and place on a heated serving platter; reserve pan liquid. Surround chicken with cooked lemon slices. Add remaining ¼ cup stock to pan liquid and cook over medium-high heat until reduced to a thin syrupy glaze. Remove from heat and blend in remaining 1 tablespoon margarine, stirring until margarine melts. Pour sauce over chicken. Makes 6 servings.

Each serving contains about:
    136 calories
    120 mg sodium
    5 g fat
    60 mg cholesterol
    Exchanges: 3 meat

CHICKEN TARRAGON

1 (3-pound) chicken
1 clove garlic, split
Pepper to taste
½ teaspoon dried tarragon, or
    2 large sprigs fresh tarragon
¾ cup low-sodium Chicken Stock (p. 40)
Tarragon Sauce (p. 198)

Rub outside and cavity of chicken with garlic. Season inside and out with pepper and sprinkle cavity with dried tarragon, or if using sprigs, place them in cavity. Moisten chicken with stock with a baster. Place chicken on rack in a roasting pan and bake at 350°F for 50 minutes to 1 hour. Remove from oven, cool slightly, and remove and discard skin. Carve and serve with Tarragon Sauce. Makes 6 servings.

Each serving with sauce contains about:
155 calories
80 mg sodium
3 g fat
60 mg cholesterol
Exchanges: 3 meat

OVEN-FRIED CHICKEN

3 whole chicken breasts (about 1½ pounds
    boned weight)
3 tablespoons egg substitute, or 1 egg
1 tablespoon water
1 teaspoon Herb Blend (p. 206)
¾ cup dry French Bread crumbs (p. 49)
2 tablespoons low-calorie margarine, melted
1 tablespoon fresh lemon juice

Skin, bone, and split chicken breasts. Pound into thin cutlets between sheets of wax paper with a mallet. Lightly beat egg substitute or egg with water. Mix Herb Blend with bread crumbs. Dip cutlets in egg mixture, then in seasoned bread crumbs. Cover and chill 1 hour.

Arrange chicken cutlets in a nonstick baking dish and drizzle each one with melted margarine and lemon juice. Bake at 350°F for 20 to 25 minutes, or until golden. Makes 6 servings.

Each serving contains about:
  182 calories
  138 mg sodium
  5 g fat
  59 mg cholesterol
  Exchanges: 3 meat, 1 bread

Turkey

TURKEY DIVAN

1 (1½-pound) turkey breast
½ pound broccoli spears, cooked
¾ cup Sauce Abel (p. 196)
Paprika
1 tablespoon minced parsley
1 tablespoon grated Parmesan cheese (optional)

Place turkey breast in a roasting pan and roast at 325°F for 40 minutes or until a meat thermometer inserted in the thickest part of breast registers 180°F. Cool slightly, then slice. Divide broccoli into 6 equal portions and arrange the portions in a nonstick baking pan. Cover each broccoli portion with a 3-ounce serving of turkey. Pour a generous tablespoon of Sauce Abel over each serving and sprinkle with paprika. Bake at 325°F for 8 minutes, or until heated through. Garnish with parsley and sprinkle with Parmesan cheese, if desired. Makes 6 servings.

Each serving with sauce and cheese contains about:
  135 calories
  113 mg sodium
  2 g fat
  72 mg cholesterol
  Exchanges: 3 meat, ½ vegetable

ROAST TURKEY WITH ROYAL GLAZE

2 tablespoons low-calorie margarine
1 cup Low-Calorie Russian Dressing (p. 183)
3 tablespoons low-calorie apricot jelly
1 (12-pound) turkey
Apple-Onion Stuffing (following recipe)

Combine margarine, Russian Dressing, and apricot jelly in a small saucepan and stir over low heat until well blended. Place turkey in a baking dish and pour marinade over. Cover and refrigerate several hours or overnight, turning occasionally. Remove turkey to roasting pan, breast side up; reserve marinade. Stuff cavity with stuffing. (Any remaining stuffing may be placed in a baking dish to bake separately at 350°F for 20 minutes.) Cover turkey loosely with foil and roast at 350°F until meat thermometer registers 180°F, basting with reserved marinade every 30 minutes. Remove foil about 20 minutes before turkey finishes roasting to brown. Makes 10 servings.

Each serving of white or dark meat contains about:
149 calories
125 mg sodium
7 g fat
72 mg cholesterol white meat; 95 mg dark meat
Exchanges: 3 low-fat meat

Apple-Onion Stuffing

2 tablespoons low-calorie margarine
1 cup chopped onions
1 shallot, minced
1 cup chopped celery
7 cups French Bread cubes (p. 49; about 14 slices)
¾ cup raisins, plumped
3 cups diced unpeeled apples
¼ cup minced parsley
1 cup chopped pecans
¼ teaspoon paprika (optional)
1¼ to 1½ cups low-sodium Turkey Stock (p. 40)

Melt the margarine in a large skillet. Add onions, shallot, and celery and sauté until onions are golden. Add bread cubes, raisins, apples, parsley, pecans, and paprika and mix well with a fork. Add just enough stock to make a moist stuffing. Use to loosely stuff turkey (½ cup per pound of bird), or place in a nonstick baking pan, cover, and bake at 350°F for 20 minutes. If stuffing dries out while baking, drizzle with more turkey stock. Makes 8 cups.

Each ¼ cup serving contains about:
74 calories
59 mg sodium
2 g fat
trace cholesterol
Exchanges: 1 bread

TURKEY TETRAZZINI

An excellent do-ahead party dish.

¼ cup low-calorie margarine
3 tablespoons flour
1½ teaspoon arrowroot
1½ teaspoon water
2½ cups low-sodium Chicken Stock (p. 40)
½ cup evaporated nonfat milk
1 (6-ounce) can low-sodium tomato paste
1 cup diced celery
4 cloves garlic, minced
½ pound mushrooms, sliced
2 cups shell macaroni, cooked
1 (1½-pound) turkey breast, or 3 chicken breasts (1½ pounds boned weight), skinned, boned, cooked, and diced
½ cup grated low-sodium Cheddar cheese

Melt margarine in a large saucepan. Add flour and stir until smooth. Dissolve arrowroot in water and stir into flour mixture until smooth. Stir in stock, milk, tomato paste, celery, garlic, and mushrooms. Cook over low heat until celery has softened slightly, about 10 minutes. Stir in cooked macaroni and turkey and turn mixture into a casserole. Cover and place in the refrigerator overnight to blend flavors. When ready to bake, remove from refrigerator, bring to room temperature, sprinkle with grated cheese and bake at 350°F for 1 hour. Makes 12 servings.

NOTE: Casserole may be covered with aluminum foil and frozen before baking. Thaw, sprinkle with cheese, and bake as directed.

Each ½ cup serving contains about:
164 calories
121 mg sodium
7 g fat
56 mg cholesterol
Exchanges: 2 meat, ¼ bread

Game

CORNISH GAME HENS
with Herb-Corn Bread Stuffing

6 Cornish game hens
1 onion, cut in 6 wedges
2 small carrots, cut in thirds
6 sprigs parsley
6 teaspoons low-calorie margarine
Pepper to taste
Herb-Corn Bread Stuffing (following recipe)

Stuff each hen cavity with an onion wedge, carrot piece, and parsley sprig. Rub 1 teaspoon margarine on each bird and sprinkle with pepper to taste. Place birds in a roasting pan and bake at 350°F for 25 minutes, or until tender. Remove from the oven. Serve with Herb-Corn Bread Stuffing. Makes 6 servings.

Each game hen (without skin) with ½ cup dressing contains about:
244 calories
128 mg sodium
6 g fat
59 mg cholesterol
Exchanges: 3 meat, 1 bread

Herb-Corn Bread Stuffing

Excellent for game birds or turkey.

> 2 tablespoons low-calorie margarine
> 1 large onion, chopped
> 3 celery stalks, chopped
> 3 cups crumbled Corn Bread (p. 47)
> 1 cup French Bread cubes (p. 49; about 1½ slices)
> 2 egg whites, lightly beaten
> ½ teaspoon pepper
> 1 teaspoon Herb Blend (p. 206)
> ¼ teaspoon freshly grated nutmeg
> 2 tablespoons sesame seeds, toasted*
> 1 cup low-sodium chicken stock

In a large skillet, melt margarine. Add onion and celery and sauté until onion is golden. Add Corn Bread, bread cubes, egg whites, pepper, Herb Blend, nutmeg, and sesame seeds and mix well. Add stock and toss gently until bread is moistened. Place stuffing in a nonstick baking dish, cover, and bake at 350°F for 20 minutes. (Or stuff fowl, allowing ½ cup stuffing for each pound.) If stuffing appears dry while baking, add a little more stock. Makes 8 servings.

*To toast sesame seeds, put them in a dry skillet and place over low heat, shaking now and then, until seeds are golden.

Each ½ cup serving contains about:
88 calories
45 mg sodium
4 g fat
trace cholesterol
Exchanges: 1 bread, ½ fat

PHEASANT UNDER GLASS

1 teaspoon vinegar
1 cup warm water
1 (2½-pound) pheasant, or 2 Cornish game hens
1 onion, cut in 4 thick slices
½ small carrot, sliced
2 sprigs parsley
3 tablespoons low-calorie margarine
Freshly ground pepper to taste
¼ cup plus 1 tablespoon low-calorie
    orange marmalade
1 tablespoon low-sodium Chicken Stock (p. 40)
2 tablespoons dry Sherry
Wild Rice Skillet (p. 133)
Watercress sprigs

Mix vinegar in water and wash neck and body cavities of pheasant with the solution. Rinse bird under running water and pat dry. (Omit this step if using game hens.) Stuff body cavity with onion and carrot slices and parsley. Rub 1 tablespoon of the margarine over the bird and sprinkle with pepper. Wrap bird in foil and place in a roasting pan. Bake at 325°F for 45 minutes.

In a small saucepan, melt remaining 2 tablespoons margarine. Remove from heat and add marmalade, stock, and Sherry, mixing well to form a glaze. Open the foil and brush the glaze over the bird. Roast 30 minutes longer, basting with pan juices. (If using Cornish game hens, reduce cooking time to 15 to 20 minutes for first roasting period and 10 minutes for second, or until tests done.) Place wild rice on a serving dish. Place bird on the rice and garnish with watercress sprigs. Carve at the table. Makes 6 servings.

Each 3 ounce serving without rice contains about:
204 calories
95 mg sodium
7 g fat
cholesterol content unavailable for pheasant
Exchanges: 3 meat

Meats

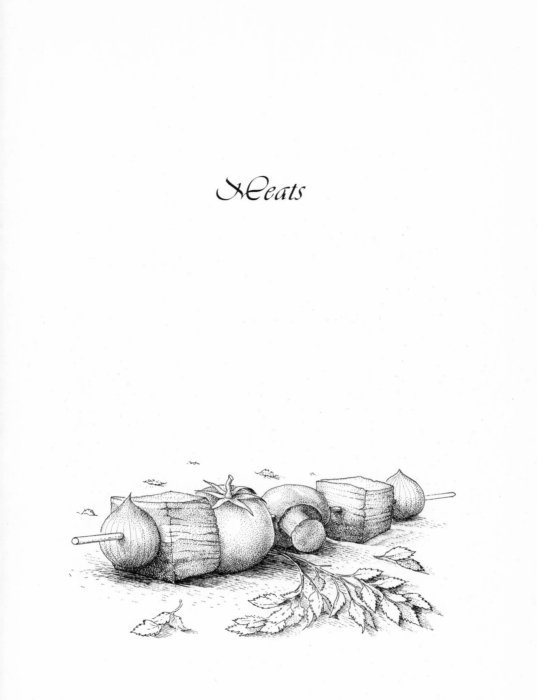

$\mathcal{A}$ll meat is an excellent source of good quality protein, niacin, iron, and thiamin. (Legumes, such as dry peas, beans, and peanuts, also are high in most of these nutrients.)

However, because the body's need for protein is limited, a little goes a long way. At best, a 3-ounce serving provides 50 percent of the RDA per serving. So, if you are concerned about fat and calories, include meat less frequently on the menu and be sure the serving sizes are limited as well. (A 3-ounce portion of meat is considered one serving.)

Some meats, however, contain higher calorie counts than others. For instance, pork, lamb, and ham are higher in calories and fat than veal and most lean beef cuts. The more marbled the beef, the higher the fat and calorie count.

Although *Light Style* recipes emphasize lower-calorie meats, there is no reason to avoid pork or lamb if you enjoy them. Simply limit portions to those recommended in the Daily Food Guide (p. 256).

Cooking methods, such as broiling, barbecuing, and simmering, will help cut calories. Trimming off any excess fat on all meats will also trim calories.

Incidentally, you will need to buy 4 ounces of raw meat to end up with 3 ounces of cooked meat, because of shrinkage during cooking. Our nutrient analysis of meat dishes allows for such shrinkage.

Beef

BEEF BROCHETTE

½ cup dry red wine
1 tablespoon Dijon Mustard (p. 203)
Pepper to taste
1½ pounds top sirloin, cut in 1-inch cubes
24 *each* cherry tomatoes, whole button mushrooms,
   and pearl onions

In a bowl, combine wine, mustard, and pepper. Add meat, cover, and refrigerate for at least 5 hours or overnight. Alternately thread meat, tomatoes, mushrooms, and onions on 6 skewers. Broil to desired doneness. Makes 6 servings.

Each serving contains about:
   211 calories
   99 mg sodium
   11 g fat
   83 mg cholesterol
   Exchanges: 3 meat

BEEF TACOS

Taco stands dot the streets of Southern California, and for good reason. People of all ages love these nutritious, easy-to-eat Mexican sandwiches. Here's a *Light Style* version.

6 corn tortillas
½ pound ground lean beef, or
   1 cup chopped cooked roast beef
½ teaspoon *each* chili powder and ground cumin
⅛ teaspoon onion powder
Pepper to taste
½ small iceberg lettuce, shredded
1 tomato, diced
6 tablespoons grated low-sodium Cheddar cheese
6 tablespoons Guacamole (p. 14)
6 tablespoons Spanish Sauce (p. 194)

Loosely fold each tortilla in half. Place a wedge of foil inside each folded tortilla to allow for filling. Secure with wood picks, if necessary. Place on a baking sheet and bake at 450°F until toasted, about 7 to 10 minutes. Discard foil and wood pick.

In a skillet, sauté ground beef with chili powder, cumin, onion powder, and pepper until browned. Gently fill openings in tortillas with 3 tablespoons *each* meat, shredded lettuce, and diced tomato, and 1 tablespoon cheese. Top each taco with 1 tablespoon *each* Guacamole and Spanish Sauce. Makes 6 servings.

Each taco contains about:
200 calories
150 mg sodium
11 g fat
42 mg cholesterol
Exchanges: ½ meat, ½ bread, ½ vegetable, 1½ fat

CHATEAUBRIAND

1 (2-pound) beef tenderloin, trimmed of fat
Garlic powder, lemon juice, and freshly ground
pepper to taste
French Provincial Sauce (p. 190)

Season tenderloin on both sides with garlic powder, lemon juice, and pepper. Place on a broiler rack and broil until meat is done as desired. Turn during broiling to cook both sides. To serve, thinly slice tenderloin on bias and arrange on a heated serving platter. Serve with French Provincial Sauce. Makes 10 servings.

Each 3 ounce serving without sauce contains about:
220 calories
56 mg sodium
11 g fat
83 mg cholesterol
Exchanges: 3 meat

CHINESE BEEF WITH PEA PODS

Serve this classic Chinese beef dish with steamed rice, broccoli, and a fruit dessert for a glamorous, yet nutritiously low-fat, low-sodium meal.

    1 tablespoon safflower oil
    4 cloves garlic, minced
1½ pounds beef tenderloin, cut into ¼-inch strips
  ¾ pound pea pods (snow peas)
    1 teaspoon grated ginger root
    2 tablespoons Soy Sauce (p. 209)
    1 tablespoon arrowroot or cornstarch
    Steamed Rice (p. 132, optional)

Heat ½ tablespoon of the oil in a hot skillet or wok until oil smokes. Add half the garlic and stir-fry 10 seconds. Add meat and stir-fry until brown. With a slotted spoon, remove meat to a bowl and set aside. Pour any juice remaining in skillet into a separate bowl and reserve. Add remaining ½ tablespoon oil to hot skillet, heat until oil smokes, and add remaining garlic. Stir-fry 10 seconds. Add pea pods and stir-fry until they turn a bright green color and are crisp but tender. Dissolve arrowroot in reserved pan juices. Push pea pods to side of skillet and add arrowroot mixture, ginger, and Soy Sauce. Cook and stir until smooth. Return meat to skillet and heat through. Serve over steamed rice, if desired. Makes 8 servings.

Each serving contains about:
233 calories
63 mg sodium
13 g fat
83 mg cholesterol
Exchanges: 3 meat, ½ B vegetable

ROAST BEEF AU JUS

1 (3- to 4-pound) sirloin tip or boned roast
Pepper to taste
3 cloves garlic, slivered
1 tablespoon low-calorie margarine
½ cup minced shallots
¾ cup dry red wine
1½ cups low-sodium Beef Stock (p. 39)
1 tablespoon minced parsley

Sprinkle roast all over with pepper. With a sharp, pointed knife blade make incisions in several places in meat and insert slivers of garlic into openings. Place in a roasting pan and roast at 325°F until meat thermometer registers 155°F for medium, or done as desired. Remove from oven. Drain pan juices and chill until surface fat coagulates, then scoop out, leaving a clear broth; set aside.

In a small skillet, melt margarine and sauté shallots until glazed but not brown. Add reserved pan juices, wine, and stock. Bring to a boil and boil until reduced by half. Stir in parsley. To serve, slice meat and spoon about 1 tablespoon sauce over each serving. Makes 10 to 12 servings.

Each 3 ounce serving with sauce contains about:
206 calories
66 mg sodium
11 g fat
83 mg cholesterol
Exchanges: 3 meat

VIENNA DIP

French Bread (p. 49)
Au jus sauce from Roast Beef au Jus (preceding recipe), heated
Thinly sliced roast beef

Slice French Bread and dip slices into sauce. Arrange beef slices on dipped slices of bread. Top each with dipped bread slice. Ladle more juice over sandwich, if desired.

Each sandwich (2 ounces meat, 2 slices bread) contains about:
292 calories
59 mg sodium
6 g fat
54 mg cholesterol
Exchanges: 2 meat, 2 bread

STEAK DIANE

6 (4-ounce) sirloin steaks or filets mignons
2 tablespoons low-calorie margarine
4 shallots, minced
1 clove garlic, minced
6 tablespoons Dijon Mustard (p. 203)
1 teaspoon chopped chives
2 tablespoons dry Sherry
¼ cup Cognac

Place the steaks between sheets of wax paper and pound with a mallet until very thin. Heat margarine in a large skillet. Add shallots and garlic and sauté until shallots are tender. Remove shallots and garlic and discard. Spread 1 tablespoon Dijon Mustard over each steak and place in skillet. Cook 3 minutes on each side. Combine chives, Sherry, and Cognac. Pour over meat and cook 1 minute longer. Makes 6 servings.

Each serving contains about:
275 calories
97 mg sodium
13 g fat
83 mg cholesterol
Exchanges: 3 meat

STEAK DIJON

¼ cup Dijon Mustard (p. 203)
½ cup dry red wine
6 (4-ounce) top sirloin or New York steaks, trimmed of fat
Freshly ground pepper to taste

Blend together mustard and wine in a small pan. Dip steaks in wine mixture and marinate, refrigerated, 1 to 2 hours. Remove steaks from marinade and broil to desired doneness, turning once. Season with pepper to taste. Makes 6 servings.

Each serving contains about:
236 calories
68 mg sodium
11 g fat
83 mg cholesterol
Exchanges: 3 meat

STEAK OSCAR

6 (4-ounce) filets mignons
12 asparagus spears, cooked (p. 138)
6 Alaskan king crab legs, 3 inches each,
   cooked and shelled
½ cup Blender Béarnaise (p. 188)
Watercress sprigs

Broil meat to desired doneness. Place 2 asparagus spears and 1 crab leg on top of each cooked filet. Pour a generous tablespoon Béarnaise Sauce over each. Garnish with watercress. Makes 6 servings.

Each serving contains about:
300 calories
92 mg sodium (content unavailable for crab)
11 g fat
103 mg cholesterol
Exchanges: 3 meat

TOURNEDOS ROSSINI

6 (4-ounce) top sirloin or tenderloin steaks
Garlic powder, lemon juice, and pepper to taste
Madeira Sauce (p. 195)

Season steaks with garlic powder, lemon juice, and pepper. Broil to desired doneness. Serve with Madeira Sauce. Makes 6 servings.

Each serving without sauce contains about:
220 calories
56 mg sodium
13 g fat
83 mg cholesterol
Exchanges: 3 meat

Lamb

IRISH STEW

1½ pounds meat from leg of lamb, cut in 1-inch cubes
1 onion, coarsely chopped
1 small turnip, cut in 1-inch cubes
2 stalks celery with some leaves, sliced
4 carrots, sliced
3 cups low-sodium Beef Stock (p. 39), or water
¼ teaspoon pepper
Bouquet Garni (p. 202)
1½ cups peeled and cubed potatoes (about 2 potatoes)
1 tablespoon cornstarch or arrowroot
1 tablespoon water
1 teaspoon Worcestershire sauce
1 tablespoon minced parsley

In a large saucepan, cook lamb cubes, onion, turnip, celery, and carrots over low heat until lamb cubes are browned. Add stock, pepper, and Bouquet Garni. Bring to a boil, reduce heat, cover and simmer for 1 hour. Add potatoes, cover, and cook 30 minutes longer, or until potatoes are tender. Dissolve cornstarch in water and stir into stew liquid. Simmer until broth is translucent. Stir in Worcestershire sauce. Sprinkle with parsley. Makes 6 servings.

Each ½ cup serving contains about:
209 calories
103 mg sodium
19 g fat
87 mg cholesterol
Exchanges: 3 meat, 1 B vegetable, ¼ bread

ROAST LEG OF LAMB WITH PINEAPPLE SAUCE

1 (3-pound) leg of lamb
4 shallots, slivered
4 cloves garlic, slivered
Juice of 1 lemon
Herb Blend (p. 206) and pepper to taste
Pineapple Sauce (p. 197)
Fresh mint sprigs

With a sharp, pointed knife blade, make incisions in several places in meat and insert slivers of shallots and garlic into openings. Squeeze lemon juice over lamb and sprinkle with Herb Blend and pepper. Roast at 325°F for 1½ to 2 hours, or until meat thermometer registers 160°F. Slice lamb and serve with Pineapple Sauce. Garnish with mint sprigs. Makes 6 servings.

Each serving without sauce contains about:
195 calories
66 mg sodium
8 g fat
92 mg cholesterol
Exchanges: 3 meat

Veal

VEAL ABEL

6 (4-ounce) veal scallops (about 1½ pounds)
2 tablespoons low-calorie margarine
½ pound mushrooms, sliced
¼ cup dry white wine
Juice of 1 lemon
Sauce Abel (p. 196)
8 asparagus spears, cooked and kept warm (p. 138)

Place veal scallops between sheets of waxed paper and pound lightly with a mallet until very thin. Melt margarine in a large skillet and sauté veal about 2 minutes on each side, or until golden brown. Remove veal and arrange on a heated platter. Add mushrooms, wine, and lemon juice to skillet and cook until mushrooms are tender, about 3 minutes. Top veal with Sauce Abel and garnish with asparagus spears and mushrooms. Makes 6 servings.

Each serving without sauce contains about:
183 calories
119 mg sodium
8 g fat
96 mg cholesterol
Exchanges: 3 meat

VEAL BOURGUIGNONNE

¼ cup low-calorie margarine
2 pounds veal rump roast, cut in 1-inch cubes
1 pound mushrooms, sliced
1 pound pearl onions, chopped
1 cup Burgundy wine
2 cups low-sodium Veal Stock
   (p. 39)
1 tablespoon dried basil
1 bay leaf
2 tablespoons arrowroot
¼ cup water

Melt margarine in a large kettle. Add veal and brown on all sides. Add mushrooms and onions and sauté until glazed. Add wine, veal stock, basil, and bay leaf. Cook over medium heat 10 minutes. Dissolve arrowroot in water, then stir into kettle. Reduce heat to a very low simmer, cover, and simmer 45 minutes, stirring often. Remove bay leaf. Makes 8 servings.
   NOTE: Lean lamb or beef may be substituted for the veal.

Each ½ cup serving contains about:
   289 calories
   150 mg sodium
   8 g fat
   115 mg cholesterol
   Exchanges: 3 meat

VEAL PARMIGIANA

6 (4-ounce) veal scallops (about 1½ pounds)
2 tablespoons low-calorie margarine
2 cups Marinara Sauce (p. 194)
6 ounces mozzarella cheese, grated
2 tablespoons grated Parmesan cheese

Place veal scallops between sheets of wax paper and pound with a mallet until very thin. Melt margarine in a large skillet and sauté veal about 2 minutes on each side, or until golden brown. Place veal in an 11-by-14-inch baking dish and top with Marinara Sauce. Sprinkle mozzarella and Parmesan cheese over sauce. Bake at 375°F for 20 minutes, or until cheese is bubbly and golden. Makes 6 servings.

Each serving contains about:
229 calories
280 mg sodium
21 g fat
95 mg cholesterol
Exchanges: 1 vegetable, 3 meat

VENETIAN VEAL

6 (4-ounce) veal scallops (about 1½ pounds)
12 sage leaves, or 1 tablespoon dried sage
2 tablespoons low-calorie margarine
½ cup dry white wine
1 teaspoon arrowroot
1 teaspoon water
Pepper to taste
2 lemons, thinly sliced

Place veal scallops between sheets of wax paper and pound with a mallet until very thin. Place a sage leaf on each side of each veal scallop and secure with a wood pick. (If using dried sage, sprinkle on both sides of each scallop.) Melt margarine in a large skillet and sauté veal 2 minutes on each side, or until golden brown. Remove veal with slotted spoon and arrange, the slices overlapping, on a heated platter. Add wine to liquid remaining in the skillet. Dissolve arrowroot in water and add to pan. Cook and stir until slightly thickened and smooth. Season with pepper. Pour sauce in a ribbon over veal and garnish with lemon slices. Makes 6 servings.

Each serving contains about:
234 calories
77 mg sodium
8 g fat
102 mg cholesterol
Exchanges: 3 meat

Pork

APPLE-STUFFED PORK CHOPS

6 (4-ounce) lean rib pork chops (about 1½ pounds)
1 tablespoon low-calorie margarine
1 tablespoon arrowroot or cornstarch
½ teaspoon maple extract
1 cup unsweetened apple juice
2 teaspoons fructose (optional)
3 small tart green apples, peeled, cored, and sliced

Have your butcher cut a pocket for stuffing in each pork chop. Melt margarine in a large skillet and brown pork chops about 3 minutes on each side. Remove and set aside. Add arrowroot, maple extract, apple juice and fructose, if desired, to saucepan. Cook over medium heat until well blended and smooth. Remove from heat and stir in apples. Cool filling slightly and stuff chops, reserving some for garnish. Secure chops with wood picks. Place chops in a baking dish, cover, and bake at 350°F for 1 hour, or until well done. Reheat any remaining filling in a small saucepan and spoon over chops to serve. Makes 6 servings.

Each chop with stuffing contains about:
319 calories
74 mg sodium
12 g fat
82 mg cholesterol
Exchanges: 3 meat, ¼ fruit

CHINESE STIR-FRY PORK

1 pound pork tenderloin
1 small onion
6 mushrooms
6 stalks celery
6 asparagus spears
2 tablespoons safflower oil
¼ cup chopped green onions
¼ teaspoon dry mustard
¼ teaspoon ground ginger
2 tablespoons Soy Sauce (p. 209)

Cut pork, onion, mushrooms, celery, and asparagus in thin julienne-style diagonal strips. Heat oil in a skillet or wok until it smokes. Add pork and stir-fry about 10 to 15 minutes. Add onion, mushrooms, celery, asparagus, green onions, mustard, and ginger, and stir-fry until vegetables are tender, about 2 to 3 minutes. Sprinkle with Soy Sauce. Makes 6 servings.

Each serving contains about:
280 calories
73 mg sodium
16 g fat
82 mg cholesterol
Exchanges: 3 meat, 1 vegetable

MEXICAN PORK STEW

You'll find the fresh tomatillos and cilantro at any Mexican market. If fresh tomatillos are not available, use small green tomatoes. Substitute Italian parsley for cilantro, if necessary. Try the tomatillo sauce with chicken, too, for a low-calorie version.

      1 tablespoon low-calorie margarine
    1½ pounds lean pork, cut in 1-inch cubes
      3 cloves garlic, minced
    1½ pounds tomatillos (Mexican green tomatoes),
          husks removed
      1 fresh jalapeño chile pepper, seeded, and chopped
      1 small onion, chopped
      ½ teaspoon fructose
      4 or 5 sprigs cilantro (fresh coriander), chopped

Melt margarine in a kettle. Add pork and garlic and sauté over medium-high heat until browned. Remove meat from pan and set aside. Place tomatillos in a saucepan with water to cover, bring to a boil, reduce heat to medium and cook, uncovered, about 5 minutes. Drain, reserving about ½ cup of the liquid. In a blender container, combine cooked tomatillos, chile pepper, onion, fructose, and blend until puréed. Pour tomatillo sauce into kettle used for browning meat and simmer for 5 minutes. Add reserved meat, cover, and simmer 45 minutes to 1 hour, or until meat is tender. Add some reserved liquid if sauce becomes too thick. Sprinkle with cilantro. Makes 8 servings.

   Each ½ cup serving contains about:
    183 calories
     66 mg sodium
     11 g fat
     51 mg cholesterol
    Exchanges: 3 meat, 1 vegetable

PORK WITH SAGE

1 (4- to 5-pound) pork loin
2 cloves garlic, slivered
2 tablespoons fresh lemon juice
1 tablespoon ground sage
Pepper to taste
Pineapple Sauce (p. 197, optional)

With a sharp, pointed knife blade, make incisions in several places in pork loin and insert slivers of garlic into the openings. Mix together lemon juice, sage, and pepper and rub mixture over pork. Place pork in a roasting pan and roast at 350°F for 35 to 45 minutes per pound, or until meat thermometer registers 185°F (about 2½ hours in all). Slice and top with Pineapple Sauce, if desired. Makes 12 servings.

Each 3 ounce serving without sauce contains about:
263 calories
60 mg sodium
11 g fat
82 mg cholesterol
Exchanges: 3 meat

Pasta and Grains

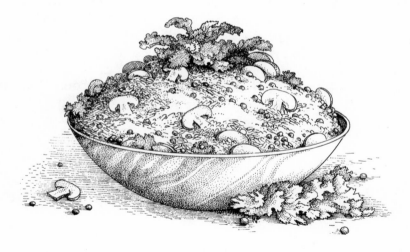

Grains, like vegetables, are known as complex carbohydrates that load the body with essential nutrients and fiber. That's why it's vitally important to include breads, cereals, and grain-based foods in your diet every day.

If you want to reduce the calories in this starchy food group, simply limit the amount of fat used to cook or season them. For example, pasta alone is not all that high in calories (only 100 calories in one-half cup cooked spaghetti). It's what you add to it that hikes the calories and makes it gloriously shameful. Cooking pasta or rice in stock will, however, eliminate the need to add more fat.

The other trick to lowering calories in rice and pasta dishes is to limit the portion size. You'll be surprised at the suggested serving size of rice and pasta recommended in the USDA Daily Food Guide on page 257. It is small enough to make you enjoy every bite!

Pasta

KATHY'S CANNELLONI

The recipe gets its name from Kathy DeKarr, a fine cook and devotee of the *Light Style* philosophy who helped us test the recipes in this book.

  1 tablespoon olive oil
½ cup minced onion
  1 teaspoon minced garlic
  1 (10-ounce) package frozen chopped spinach,
     thawed and drained
  1 teaspoon low-calorie margarine
½ pound ground lean beef
  1 chicken liver
  2 tablespoons plus 1 teaspoon grated
     Parmesan cheese
  1 tablespoon evaporated nonfat milk
  3 tablespoons egg substitute, or 1 egg
1¼ teaspoons dried oregano
   Pepper to taste
18 Cannelloni Noodles (recipe following)
  1 cup Marinara Sauce (p. 194)
¾ cup Béchamel Sauce (p. 187)

Heat oil in a skillet and add onion and garlic. Sauté over medium-high heat until onion is golden and tender. Stir in spinach. Cook and stir 3 to 4 minutes, or until all the moisture has evaporated. Transfer the spinach mixture to a large bowl. In the same skillet, melt ½ teaspoon of the margarine. Add beef and cook until lightly browned. Add beef mixture to spinach mixture. Melt remaining ½ teaspoon margarine in the same skillet and add the chicken liver. Cook for 3 to 4 minutes, or until liver is firm and browned on all sides. Chop liver coarsely and add to spinach-beef mixture. Then add 2 tablespoons of the Parmesan cheese, milk, egg substitute or egg, oregano, and pepper and mix well. Place 1 tablespoon of the filling on the unbrowned side of each Cannelloni Noodle. Fold sides over filling so

Pasta and Grains   125

they overlap and tuck in ends. Repeat until all crêpes are filled and folded. Pour a thin layer of Marinara Sauce in a shallow 14-by-10-inch baking pan. Arrange cannelloni in a single layer over sauce. Pour Béchamel Sauce over cannelloni and spoon remaining Marinara Sauce on top. Sprinkle with remaining cheese and bake, uncovered, at 375°F for 20 minutes. Place under broiler 30 seconds to brown top. Makes 18 cannelloni.

Each cannelloni contains about:
75 calories
78 mg sodium
5 g fat
21 mg cholesterol
Exchanges: ½ meat, ½ bread

Cannelloni Noodles

Make these low-calorie, low-fat crêpes ahead and stack between sheets of wax paper in the refrigerator or freezer to use with fillings and toppings of your choice.

½ cup unbleached flour
½ cup water
¾ cup egg substitute, or 2 eggs
2 teaspoons low-calorie margarine

Combine flour, water, and egg substitute or eggs and beat with a rotary beater or wire whisk until well blended. Chill batter. Heat a 5-inch skillet or crêpe pan until very hot and brush lightly with some of the margarine. Remove from heat and pour in about 1 tablespoon batter. Lift and tilt pan to evenly spread batter over pan bottom. Return to heat and cook until crêpe is lightly browned on underside. Turn and cook about 5 seconds, then remove to wax paper. (Crêpe should *not* brown; it should remain pale.) Repeat until all batter is used, lightly greasing the pan occasionally. Makes 18.

Each cannelloni noodle contains about:
22 calories
20 mg sodium
2 g fat
0 mg cholesterol
Exchanges: ½ bread

FETTUCCINI ALFREDO

8 ounces dry fettuccini noodles
2 quarts low-sodium Chicken Stock, (p. 40)
½ cup low-calorie sour cream
½ cup low-fat plain yogurt
2 tablespoons low-calorie margarine
2 cloves garlic, minced
3 tablespoons chopped parsley
1 tablespoon poppy seeds
2 tablespoons grated Parmesan cheese (optional)

Cook noodles in boiling stock until tender but firm to the bite, about 12 minutes. Drain and set aside. In a small bowl, mix together sour cream and yogurt until smooth; set aside. Melt margarine in a large skillet and sauté garlic 1 minute. Reduce heat to low and add yogurt mixture, blending well. Add noodles and toss gently until sauce is evenly distributed. Sprinkle with parsley, poppy seeds, and Parmesan cheese, if desired. Makes 8 servings.

Each ½ cup serving with cheese contains about:
132 calories
62 mg sodium
5 g fat
36 mg cholesterol
Exchanges: 1 bread, 1 fat

LASAGNA

This lasagna goes light on fats and starch to help lower the calories.

8 ounces lasagna noodles
1 pound ricotta cheese (made from
    partially skimmed milk)
6 tablespoons egg substitute, or 2 eggs
⅛ teaspoon ground nutmeg
2 tablespoons minced parsley
3 cups Italian Meat Sauce (p. 192)
1 pound mozzarella cheese, shredded
½ cup grated Parmesan cheese (optional)

Cook lasagna until just tender. Drain, rinse, and let stand in cold water. Beat ricotta cheese with egg substitute or eggs. Stir in nutmeg and parsley. Cover the bottom of a 9-by-13-inch nonstick baking pan with a ¼-inch layer of Italian Meat Sauce. Top with a layer of half the noodles and add half of the remaining meat sauce. Spread half of the ricotta cheese mixture over meat sauce and sprinkle with half of the mozzarella cheese. Repeat layers, ending with mozzarella cheese. Sprinkle evenly with Parmesan cheese if desired, and bake at 375°F for 35 minutes, or until cheese melts and is golden. Makes 16 servings.

Each 2-by-3-inch piece with Parmesan cheese contains about:
257 calories
264 mg sodium
12 g fat
53 mg cholesterol (content unavailable for lasagna noodles)
Exchanges: 1 vegetable, 3 meat, ½ bread

NOODLES SIMPLICE

2 quarts low-sodium Chicken Stock (p. 40)
8 ounces dry noodles
2 tablespoons low-calorie margarine
2 cloves garlic, minced
2 tablespoons chopped parsley

Bring stock to a boil in a large pot. Add noodles and cook until tender but firm to the bite, about 8 minutes. Drain and place on a heated platter. Melt margarine in a small saucepan and stir in garlic and parsley. Heat gently. Pour parsley mixture over noodles and toss to coat well. Makes 8 servings.

Each ½ cup serving contains about:
112 calories
24 mg sodium
3 g fat
25 mg cholesterol (with egg noodles; trace, plain noodles)
Exchanges: 1 bread

SPAGHETTI WITH ITALIAN MEAT SAUCE

    1 quart *each* water and low-sodium Chicken Stock, (p. 40)
    8 ounces spaghetti
 1½ cups Italian Meat Sauce (p. 192), heated
    2 tablespoons grated Parmesan cheese (optional)

Place water and chicken stock in a large pot and bring to a boil. Add spaghetti and cook until tender but firm to the bite, about 10 minutes; drain. Place spaghetti in a heated serving platter or bowl. Spoon Italian Meat Sauce over spaghetti and toss quickly until well coated. Sprinkle with cheese if desired. Makes 6 to 8 servings.

 Each ½ cup serving with cheese contains about:
 150 calories
 58 mg sodium
 3 g fat
 32 mg cholesterol
 Exchanges: 1 bread, 1 meat

Rice

CONFETTI RICE

    2 cups low-sodium Beef Stock (p. 39), or
        Chicken Stock (p. 40)
    1 cup long-grain rice
    2 tablespoons low-calorie margarine
 10 mushrooms, sliced
 ½ cup frozen petite peas, thawed, or fresh shelled peas
    2 tablespoons chopped parsley

Bring stock to a boil in a saucepan. Add rice and 1 tablespoon of the margarine and bring again to a boil. Stir, cover, reduce heat to low, and cook for 25 minutes or until rice is tender and moisture is absorbed.

 Just before rice is cooked, melt remaining 1 tablespoon margarine in a skillet. Add mushrooms and sauté over high heat until almost tender and liquid has evaporated, stirring frequently. Add peas and toss with mushrooms until peas are hot. Add mushroom mixture and parsley to cooked rice. Toss lightly to mix. Makes 6 servings.

Each ½ cup serving contains about:
80 calories
52 mg sodium
3 g fat
1 mg cholesterol
Exchanges: 1 bread

RICE PILAF

2½ cups low-sodium chicken stock
1½ cups unsweetened apple juice
¼ cup wild rice
1 cup long-grain rice
1 tablespoon low-calorie margarine

Bring stock and apple juice to a boil in a saucepan. Add wild rice and bring again to a boil. Reduce heat to low, cover, and cook for 15 minutes. Add long-grain rice, cover, and continue to cook for 30 minutes, or until rice is tender and moisture is absorbed. Turn into a serving bowl and fluff with a fork. Add margarine to rice and toss lightly. Makes 6 servings.

Each ½ cup serving contains about:
102 calories
13 mg sodium
2 g fat
trace cholesterol
Exchanges: 1 bread

SAFFRON RICE

1 teaspoon low-calorie margarine
½ medium onion, finely chopped
1 clove garlic, minced
2 cups low-sodium Chicken Stock (p. 40)
1 cup long-grain rice
Pinch saffron threads

In a saucepan, melt margarine and add onion and garlic. Sauté until onion is tender and golden. Add stock, bring to a boil, and add rice and saffron. Bring again to a boil, stir, cover, reduce heat to low, and cook 25 minutes or until rice is tender and moisture is absorbed. Makes 6 servings.

Each ½-cup serving contains about:
80 calories
8 mg sodium
trace fat
trace cholesterol
Exchanges: 1 bread

SPANISH RICE

2 cups low-sodium Chicken Stock, (p. 40)
½ cup low-sodium tomato purée*
1 tablespoon vegetable oil
1 small onion, chopped
1 small green pepper, minced
1 cup long-grain rice

Combine stock, tomato purée, and oil in a saucepan. Bring to a boil and stir in onion, green pepper, and rice. Bring again to a boil, reduce heat, cover, and cook 25 minutes or until rice is tender and moisture is absorbed. Makes 8 servings.

*To make your own low-sodium tomato purée, place fresh peeled tomatoes or low-sodium canned tomatoes in a blender container and blend until smooth.

Each ½ cup serving contains about:
  107 calories
  7 mg sodium
  2 g fat
  trace cholesterol
  Exchanges: 1 bread

STEAMED RICE

2 cups low-sodium Chicken Stock, (p. 40)
1 cup long-grain rice
1 tablespoon low-calorie margarine

Bring stock to a boil in a saucepan. Add rice and bring again to a boil. Reduce heat to low, cover, and cook 25 minutes, or until rice is tender and moisture is absorbed. Turn into a serving bowl and fluff with a fork. Add margarine and toss lightly. Makes 6 servings.

Each ½ cup serving contains about:
  95 calories
  26 mg sodium
  1 g fat
  trace cholesterol
  Exchanges: 1 bread

WILD RICE SKILLET

Wild rice is loaded with nutrients. It is difficult to harvest, however, which keeps it a luxury. You can stretch pennies and taste by combining cooked wild rice with white or brown rice. Just remember that 1 cup of uncooked wild rice will yield about 3 cups cooked.

    4 cups low-sodium Chicken Stock (p. 40; or amount
        specified in wild rice package directions)
    1 cup wild rice
 1½ tablespoons low-calorie margarine
    1 clove garlic, pressed
    ¼ pound mushrooms, thinly sliced
    6 water chestnuts, sliced
    2 tablespoons slivered almonds
    Minced parsley

Bring stock to a boil in a saucepan. Add rice, reduce heat to low, cover, and cook about 60 minutes, or until rice is tender and moisture is absorbed. Melt margarine in a large skillet and add garlic and mushrooms. Sauté until mushrooms are almost tender, about 3 minutes. Add water chestnuts and almonds and sauté 1 minute longer, or until mushrooms are tender. Add rice and toss lightly. Sprinkle with parsley. Makes 6 servings.

    Each ½ cup serving contains about:
    105 calories
    38 mg sodium
    3 g fat
    trace cholesterol
    Exchanges: 1 bread, ¼ fat

Vegetables

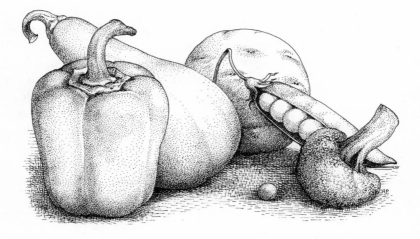

$\mathcal{T}$hey are called complex carbohydrates and nutritionists recommend eating more of them.

Vegetables are especially high in vitamins C and A. Vitamin C (ascorbic acid) plays an important role in the repair and growth of all body tissues, bones, and teeth. Because vitamin C is water soluble and not stored by the body, it is necessary to eat good sources each day in the form of fruits and vegetables. Broccoli, cantaloupe, collard greens, Brussels sprouts, strawberries, and oranges and other citrus fruits are especially high in vitamin C.

Vitamin A helps build body cells and is essential in children's growth and in the development of fetuses. Adequate supplies of vitamin A in the diet assure healthy bones and skin. Vitamin A occurs as retinol, a chemical found in foods of animal sources, and carotene, an orange plant pigment. Both are fat soluble. Carotene, which is converted to vitamin A in the body, is found in carrots, sweet potatoes, and other yellow and some red and dark-green leafy vegetables. Dark-green leafy or orange vegetables should be included in the diet three or four times a week. Teenagers will derive extra sources of riboflavin and calcium needed for growing bones and body tissue from broccoli and other dark-green leafy vegetables.

Vegetables also contain fiber, which helps in regular elimination. Ideally, everyone should have four vegetable servings each day. A typical vegetable serving is only ½ cup.

So permit us to present the *Light Style* approach to vegetables. Our recipes are even lower in calories, cholesterol, fats, and salt than you would expect. Of course, fresh vegetables are preferred to frozen or canned vegetable products.

You'll find a few simple, yet flavorful, vegetable dishes among fancy ones. Complementary use of spices and herbs all but eliminates the need for salt. All the sauces used with vegetables are de-

136

signed to be as low in calories as possible. We use minimal amounts of fats and substitute arrowroot for flour when thickening to help reduce total calories or fats.

Vegetables are not only beautiful and naturally tasty, they are easy and quick to prepare. In fact, fresh vegetables often take as little time as it would take to heat a frozen-food packet or canned product.

Vegetables, however, like any fragile food, lose vitamins and minerals, texture, color, and flavor value when overcooked or cooked in too much water. Nutrients and flavor also deteriorate when vegetables are stored too long or improperly.

If you are cooking vegetables on the stove, steam them, preferably on a steamer rack to keep them out of the water to best preserve nutrients. You'll preserve further nutrients by covering the pot during any type of cooking. Do not cook the vegetables too long or you will damage color along with nutrients. If you cook vegetables in water, reserve it for use in sauces, soups, and stocks.

Stir-frying is also a good cooking method for preserving nutrients and enhancing flavor. The Chinese method of rapid cooking over high heat just until color heightens and vegetables are crisp but tender helps preserve the best characteristics of vegetables. (A little oil, sometimes wine or broth, can be used to keep the vegetables from sticking or scorching when stir-frying.) Be cautious: Exposure to high heat for a long time will destroy anything, including vegetables.

Microwave cooking, according to the latest information we have, best preserves nutrients, texture, and color of most vegetables, especially those requiring no cooking liquid, such as baked potatoes.

Choose vegetables that look healthy and have good color. If the vegetables are shriveled or bruised, don't buy them. Fresh vegetables store well in the refrigerator for up to a week. Root vegetables can be stored in a cool, dry place away from light for several weeks. All vegetables should be used as soon after purchase as possible.

STEAMING VEGETABLES

Cut vegetables as desired or leave whole. Place in a steamer rack or colander that fits a deep pot. Place rack in pot and add enough water to fill bottom without touching steamer rack, about 1½ inches. Cover and cook at medium-high heat until vegetables reach a high color and are tender but crisp. Cooking time will depend on variety and size of vegetable. Remove vegetables to serving bowl or platter and season as desired. Reserve steaming liquid for use in sauces, soups, and stocks. Vegetables that stand too long after cooking deteriorate in vitamin and mineral content.

STEAMED ASPARAGUS

1½ pounds asparagus spears
1 tablespoon low-calorie margarine
1 teaspoon dried marjoram

Trim woody ends of asparagus spears. Steam asparagus according to preceding directions for about 5 to 7 minutes. Drain. Melt margarine in a small saucepan and stir in marjoram. Pour over asparagus. Makes 6 servings.

NOTE: For a more elaborate dish, add 1 tablespoon sesame seeds to the margarine-marjoram mixture and sauté until golden. Then add 2 tablespoons fresh lemon juice and heat through. Nutrient Analysis: 33 calories; 13 mg sodium; 2 g fat.

Each serving (4 spears) contains about:
20 calories
19 mg sodium
1 g fat
0 mg cholesterol
Exchanges: 1 vegetable

Asparagus Picante

Prepare Steamed Asparagus as in preceding recipe. Add to margarine-marjoram mixture 2 tablespoons fresh lemon juice and 1 tablespoon each mild sesame oil and white wine vinegar. Sprinkle with chopped cilantro (fresh coriander).

Each serving (4 spears) contains about:
40 calories
19 mg sodium
3 g fat
0 mg cholesterol
Exchanges: 1 vegetable

BROCCOLI ALLA ROMANA

1 tablespoon safflower oil
1 teaspoon finely chopped garlic
3 cups broccoli flowerets (about 2 pounds broccoli)
Pepper to taste
Juice of 1 lemon
6 tablespoons Mock Hollandaise (p. 201, optional)

Heat oil in a skillet or wok. Add garlic and cook for 30 seconds. Add broccoli flowerets and toss until tender, but crisp (about 7 minutes). With a slotted spoon, transfer flowerets to a heated bowl and sprinkle with pepper and lemon juice. If desired, top each serving with 1 tablespoon Mock Hollandaise. Makes 6 servings.

Each ½ cup serving without sauce contains about:
40 calories
19 mg sodium
2 g fat
0 mg cholesterol
Exchanges: 1 vegetable, ¼ fat

CARROTS A L'ORANGE

1½ pounds carrots, peeled and thinly sliced
4½ teaspoons low-calorie orange marmalade
1 teaspoon low-calorie margarine
Dash ground nutmeg

Cook carrots according to directions for Steaming Vegetables (page 137). When almost tender (about 7 to 10 minutes), drain carrots and place in a skillet. Add marmalade, margarine, and nutmeg to skillet and cook, stirring occasionally, until carrots are glazed. Makes 6 servings.

Each ½ cup serving contains about:
35 calories
61 mg sodium

trace fat
0 mg cholesterol
Exchanges: 1 vegetable

CAULIFLOWER IN LEMON SAUCE

1 medium head cauliflower
1½ cups low-fat milk
2 tablespoons low-calorie margarine
2 cloves garlic, finely minced
2 tablespoons chopped parsley
2 teaspoons fresh lemon juice

Cut off tough end of cauliflower stem and remove any leaves. Place whole cauliflower upright in a saucepan, add milk, and bring just to a boil. (The milk will prevent discoloration.) Reduce heat and simmer, partially covered, until the stalk is just tender, about 15 to 20 minutes. Drain and place cauliflower in a serving dish. Melt margarine in a small saucepan and add garlic, parsley, and lemon juice. Mix well and pour over cauliflower. Makes 6 servings.

Each ½ cup serving contains about:
32 calories
42 mg sodium
2 g fat
0 mg cholesterol
Exchanges: 1 vegetable, ¼ fat

CHINESE STIR-FRY VEGETABLES

½ cup low-sodium Beef Stock (p. 39)
2 tablespoons minced ginger root
¼ head cauliflower, broken into flowerets
¼ pound broccoli, broken into flowerets
½ cup julienne-cut celery
¼ pound pea pods (snow peas)
¼ head Napa cabbage, shredded
10 mushrooms, diced
¼ pound bamboo shoots, diced
1 tablespoon Soy Sauce (p. 209)
½ cup water chestnuts, thinly sliced
1 medium onion, thinly sliced
¼ pound bean sprouts

Heat stock in a heated wok or skillet. Add ginger root, cauliflowerets, broccoli, celery, and pea pods. Stir-fry 2 minutes over high heat. Add cabbage, mushrooms, and bamboo shoots. Stir-fry 1 minute. Stir in Soy Sauce and simmer over low heat 1 minute. Add water chestnuts, onion, and bean sprouts and stir-fry 1 minute over high heat. Do not overcook; vegetables should be tender but crisp. Makes 10 servings.

Each ½ cup serving contains about:
41 calories
33 mg sodium
trace fat
0 mg cholesterol
Exchanges: 1 vegetable

CREAMED SPINACH

½ cup water
2 pounds fresh spinach, trimmed, or
    2 (10-ounce) packages frozen chopped spinach
1 tablespoon low-calorie margarine
1½ tablespoons flour
¼ cup nonfat milk
¼ cup evaporated skim milk
¼ teaspoon ground nutmeg
Dash onion powder

Heat water in a large skillet, add spinach, cover, and cook over high heat until steam appears. Reduce heat and simmer until tender, about 5 minutes. Drain and chop spinach; set aside. (If using frozen spinach, cook according to package directions, omitting salt; drain well.)

In a small saucepan, melt margarine, add flour, and stir until smooth. Slowly add milks, stirring continually to make a smooth sauce. Bring to a boil, reduce heat, and simmer for 1 minute, stirring constantly. Sauce will be very thick. Remove from heat and season with nutmeg and onion powder. Mix the sauce with the spinach until evenly blended. Makes 6 servings.

Each ½ cup serving contains about:
66 calories
24 mg sodium
1 g fat
2 mg cholesterol
Exchanges: ½ bread

GREEN BEANS AMANDINE

1½ pounds green beans, trimmed
½ cup low-sodium Chicken Stock (p. 40)
1 tablespoon low-calorie margarine
2 cloves garlic, minced
¼ cup slivered almonds
1 tablespoon chopped shallots, or
    1 small onion, chopped

Sliver (French cut) beans or leave them whole. Place in a skillet with stock, bring to a boil, reduce heat, cover, and cook until beans are tender, about 5 to 7 minutes for French cut or about 10 to 15 minutes for whole beans. Drain beans and place on a heated platter. Melt margarine in skillet and add garlic, almonds, and shallots. Sauté until shallots are glazed and golden; do not brown. Add to beans and toss to coat well. Makes 6 servings.

Each ½ cup serving contains about:
    40 calories
    27 mg sodium
    1 g fat
    0 mg cholesterol
    Exchanges: 1 vegetable

HERBED CROOKNECK SQUASH

6 small crookneck squash (about 1 pound), trimmed
1 teaspoon dried basil
¼ teaspoon *each* onion powder and garlic powder
Pepper to taste
Low-sodium Chicken Stock (p. 40)

Cut squash in half lengthwise. Place squash, basil, onion and garlic powders and pepper in a skillet with 1-inch stock. Cover and cook 7 to 8 minutes, or until squash is crisp but tender. Remove with a slotted spoon to a heated serving platter. Makes 6 servings.

Each ½ cup serving contains about:
    19 calories
    3 mg sodium
    0 g fat
    0 mg cholesterol
    Exchanges: 1 vegetable

LEMON SPINACH

1 tablespoon low-calorie margarine
2 cloves garlic, minced
¼ cup water (if using fresh spinach)
2 pounds fresh spinach, trimmed, or
      2 (10-ounce) packages frozen chopped spinach
Juice of 1 large lemon
Lemon wedges

Melt margarine in a skillet, add garlic, and sauté 1 minute. Add water and spinach, cover, and simmer 2 to 3 minutes, or until spinach is tender. Drain off excess liquid. (If using frozen spinach, cook according to package directions, omitting salt. Add, without water, to sautéed garlic and heat through.) Turn spinach into serving plate. Sprinkle with lemon juice and garnish with lemon wedges. Makes 6 servings.

Each ½ cup serving contains about:
26 calories
27 mg sodium
trace fat
0 mg cholesterol
Exchanges: 1 vegetable

MINTED BABY CARROTS

1½ pounds small carrots, peeled
1 tablespoon low-calorie margarine
2 tablespoons fresh lemon juice
2 tablespoons chopped fresh mint

Cook carrots according to directions for Steaming Vegetables (page 137). Drain. Melt margarine in a small saucepan and stir in lemon juice. Add carrots and toss to coat well. Place on a serving platter and sprinkle with mint. Makes 6 servings.

Each ½ cup serving contains about:
32 calories
62 mg sodium

1 g fat
0 mg cholesterol
Exchanges: 1 vegetable

MUSHROOM SAUTE

An excellent flavor complement for beef, veal, or chicken.

1 tablespoon low-calorie margarine
1 pound mushrooms, sliced
2 tablespoons chopped shallots
3 tablespoons dry red wine
2 tablespoons minced parsley

Melt margarine in a large skillet and add mushrooms and shallots. Sauté until shallots are glazed and mushrooms are tender. Add wine and cook until juices reduce slightly, about 2 to 3 minutes. Stir in parsley. Makes 6 servings.

Each ½ cup serving contains about:
24 calories
24 mg sodium
1 g fat
0 mg cholesterol
Exchanges: 1 vegetable

PEAS AND PODS

High in calories and nutrients, too.

Romaine lettuce leaves
1½ pounds fresh peas, shelled, or
    2 (10-ounce) packages frozen peas
1 pound fresh pea pods (snow peas), or
    1 (10-ounce) package frozen pea pods
4 green onions, thinly sliced
2 tablespoons minced celery leaves
½ teaspoon dried rosemary
Pepper to taste

Line a heavy skillet with 3 large lettuce leaves. Place peas and pea pods on lettuce leaves. Sprinkle with green onions, celery leaves, rosemary, and pepper. Top with another layer of lettuce leaves. Tightly cover and cook over medium heat 10 to 12 minutes, or until tender. Do not overcook or peas will stick to pan bottom. Cut up cooked lettuce leaves and serve with peas, if desired. Makes 8 servings.

NOTE: Those on an extremely low sodium-restricted diet should use fresh peas and pea pods.

Each ½ cup serving contains about:
60 calories
3 mg sodium (115 mg if using frozen peas)
trace fat
0 mg cholesterol
Exchanges: 1 B vegetable

RATATOUILLE

An excellent low-fat, no-cholesterol accompaniment to meats.

1 tablespoon olive oil or safflower oil
6 green onions, chopped
6 small zucchini, thinly sliced
4 cloves garlic, minced
Pepper to taste
1 medium eggplant, diced
1 small green bell pepper, chopped
3 tomatoes, peeled and chopped
2 teaspoons dried basil, or
   2 tablespoons chopped fresh basil
1 teaspoon dried oregano, or
   1 tablespoon chopped fresh oregano
2 tablespoons chopped parsley

Using a Dutch oven or flameproof casserole, heat oil and add onions, zucchini, garlic, and pepper. Sauté for 2 minutes, stirring constantly. Add eggplant, green pepper, tomatoes, basil, and oregano. Cover and simmer 10 minutes. Remove cover and simmer until juices are reduced and thickened. Sprinkle with parsley. Serve hot or cold. Makes 6 servings.

Each ½ cup serving contains about:
22 calories
3 mg sodium
trace fat
0 mg cholesterol
Exchanges: 1 vegetable

SAVORY GREEN BEANS

1¼ **pounds green beans, trimmed**
½ **cup low-sodium Chicken Stock (p. 40)**
1 **tablespoon low-calorie margarine**
½ **teaspoon dill weed or 1 fresh sprig dill, minced**
¾ **teaspoon dried marjoram or summer savory**
Lemon wedges

Cut beans on the diagonal into 1½-inch slices. Cook green beans in stock until tender. Drain and arrange on a heated platter. In a saucepan, melt margarine and add dill and marjoram. Spoon herb-margarine mixture over green beans and toss gently. Garnish with lemon wedges. Makes 6 servings.

Each ½ cup serving contains about:
25 calories
28 mg sodium
1 g fat
trace cholesterol
Exchanges: 1 vegetable

SHREDDED ZUCCHINI

2 pounds zucchini or pattypan squash, trimmed
¼ cup chopped parsley
2 cloves garlic, minced
1 tablespoon low-calorie margarine
6 green onions, chopped
Pepper to taste
2 tablespoons grated Parmesan cheese (optional)

Shred the squash. Place in a tea towel and squeeze out excess moisture. In a skillet, combine the squash, parsley, garlic, margarine, onions, and pepper. Cover and cook over low heat 2 minutes. Uncover and raise heat to medium-high to reduce liquid in pan. To serve, sprinkle with cheese, if desired. Makes 6 servings.

Each ½ cup serving without cheese contains about:
17 calories
19 mg sodium
1 g fat
0 mg cholesterol
Exchanges: 1 vegetable

WHIPPED BUTTERNUT SQUASH

1 (1½-pound) butternut squash
2 tablespoons low-calorie margarine
1 teaspoon fructose
¼ teaspoon ground cinnamon
Dash ground allspice
¼ cup unsweetened orange juice

Place squash on an oven rack. Bake at 375°F until it can be pierced easily with a wood pick, about 1 hour. Cut in half and remove and discard seeds. Scoop out flesh and mash. Add margarine, fructose, cinnamon, allspice, and orange juice and beat until smooth. Makes 6 servings.

Each ½ cup serving contains about:
  62 calories
  25 mg sodium
  1 g fat
  0 mg cholesterol
  Exchanges: 1 vegetable

ZUCCHINI OREGANO

1½ pounds zucchini, sliced
1 large tomato, chopped
2 tablespoons minced shallots or green onions
      (white part only)
1 tablespoon fresh lemon juice
1½ teaspoons chopped fresh oregano, or
      ½ teaspoon dried oregano
1 tablespoon chopped parsley
Pepper to taste

Place zucchini, tomato, and shallots in a skillet. Cover and cook over low heat until zucchini is crisp, but tender. Place in a heated serving dish. In a small bowl, combine lemon juice, oregano, parsley, and pepper. Pour over zucchini mixture and mix gently. Makes 6 servings.

Each ½ cup serving contains about:
  13 calories
  2 mg sodium
  0 g fat
  0 mg cholesterol
  Exchanges: 1 vegetable

Potatoes

CANDIED SWEETS

An excellent source of vitamin A and fiber.

    3 medium sweet potatoes
1½ tablespoons low-calorie margarine
1½ teaspoons cornstarch
    1 teaspoon fructose
    ⅛ teaspoon maple extract
    ½ cup unsweetened pineapple juice

Cook sweet potatoes in boiling water to cover until almost tender, about 20 minutes. Peel and cut lengthwise in ½-inch slices. Put the slices in a baking dish and set aside. Dissolve cornstarch, fructose and maple extract in pineapple juice in a small saucepan. Cook and stir until smooth and thickened. Spoon glaze over potatoes. Bake at 375°F for about 20 minutes. Makes 6 servings.

Each ½ cup serving contains about:
81 calories
20 mg sodium
2 g fat
0 mg cholesterol
Exchanges: 1 bread

CHANTILLY POTATOES

3½ cups boiling water
1 small onion, or 1 clove garlic, split
1 bay leaf
Celery leaves from 1 stalk celery
3 medium potatoes (about 1½ pounds),
    peeled and quartered
¼ cup low-fat milk
¼ cup low-calorie sour cream
2 tablespoons low-calorie margarine
1 tablespoon minced chives
⅛ teaspoon *each* onion powder and garlic powder
Pepper to taste
⅛ teaspoon paprika

Combine water, onion, bay leaf, and celery leaves in a large kettle. Bring to a boil, add potatoes, and cook, covered, until potatoes are tender, about 25 to 35 minutes. Remove and mash potatoes. Add milk, sour cream, and margarine to potatoes and beat until creamy. Blend in chives, onion powder, garlic powder, and pepper. To fluff mashed potatoes, cover the pan and place over very low heat about 5 minutes. Sprinkle with paprika. Makes 6 servings.

Each ½ cup serving contains about:
  89 calories
  56 mg sodium
  4 g fat
  5 mg cholesterol
  Exchanges: ½ bread, 1 fat

OVEN-FRIED POTATOES

You'll reserve nutrients and fiber if you don't peel.

3 medium potatoes, peeled or unpeeled
3½ tablespoons low-calorie margarine, melted
Paprika

Cut potatoes lengthwise into strips about 4-by-½-by-¼ inches. Arrange in a single layer on a baking sheet. Pour margarine over potatoes, and toss to coat well. Sprinkle with paprika. Bake at 450°F for 30 to 40 minutes, tossing several times during baking. Drain on paper toweling. Makes 6 servings.

Each serving (½ potato) contains about:
83 calories
65 mg sodium
3 g fat
0 mg cholesterol
Exchanges: ½ bread, ½ fat

POMMES PARISIENNE

24 small new red potatoes
3 tablespoons low-calorie margarine
3 tablespoons chopped parsley, dill, or chives

Peel a thin strip of skin from around the center of each potato. Place potatoes in 1 inch of water in a saucepan. Bring to a boil, cover, reduce heat, and simmer until tender, about 25 minutes. Drain. Melt margarine in a saucepan over low heat and add potatoes. Shake pan gently until potatoes are well coated. Sprinkle with parsley. Makes 6 servings.

Each serving (4 potatoes) contains about:
71 calories
56 mg sodium
3 g fat
0 mg cholesterol
Exchanges: 1 bread, ½ fat

STUFFED BAKED POTATOES

3 (6-ounce) baking potatoes
4 tablespoons evaporated nonfat milk
¼ cup low-calorie sour cream
2 tablespoons low-calorie margarine
Dash ground nutmeg
1 tablespoon chopped chives
1 teaspoon fresh lemon juice
Pepper to taste
3 egg whites
1 teaspoon white vinegar
Paprika

Pierce potatoes with fork to allow steam to escape during cooking. Bake at 400°F until tender when pierced with a fork, 45 minutes to 1 hour. Cut potatoes in half lengthwise and scoop out pulp, leaving skins intact. Mash pulp and blend in milk, sour cream, margarine, nutmeg, chives, lemon juice, and pepper. Whip until smooth. Place egg whites in a bowl, add vinegar, and beat until stiff. Fold into whipped potato mixture. Mound potato mixture in reserved skins with a spoon (or use a pastry bag) and sprinkle with paprika. Place in a baking dish and bake at 375°F for 10 minutes. Makes 6 servings.

Each serving contains about:
93 calories
50 mg sodium
4 g fat
1 mg cholesterol
Exchanges: 1 bread, 1 fat

Salads

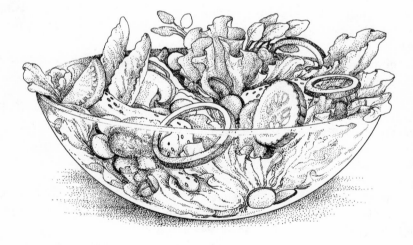

$\mathcal{T}$he New American Cuisine dictates abundant use of salads because they are naturally light and naturally nutritious. They also are beautiful to look at and simple to prepare— important features of the *Light Style* approach to dining.

You really don't have to do too much to make salads conform to *Light Style* eating, but we have taken steps to trim calories, fats, and cholesterol even further and have done away with salt.

The tricks we employ can be applied to your own salad making. Low-calorie mayonnaise (imitation mayonnaise contains no cholesterol and less fat than regular, not fake ingredients), low-fat dairy products, such as low-fat yogurt and sour cream, and evaporated nonfat milk, and unsweetened fruit juices help cut calories and reduce cholesterol. Weight worriers, in fact, will get top calorie mileage by eating salads. Plus, low-sodium cheese will help you reduce sodium intake.

Ingenious use of herbs and spices all but obviates the need for salt, as you will see for yourself when preparing these or your own salad with herb concoctions.

Salads are a wonderful source of complex carbohydrates, ready to contribute their share of nutrients to your total daily account if you choose nutrient-dense fruits and vegetables. They also are good sources of fiber. A variety approach will insure intake of trace minerals that may be missing otherwise.

Choose dark-green leafy vegetables for their high nutrient value. Parsley is not only a convenient garnish but an iron-rich vegetable high in vitamin C, too. Watercress is a good source of vitamin A. Spinach is loaded with iron and other fine nutrients. (A half-cup serving of fresh spinach provides almost twice the amount of vitamin A and half the vitamin C needed each day.)

Fruits contribute varying degrees of calories, but almost all of them contribute valuable nutrients. Strawberries, citrus fruits, and

156

cantaloupe, for instance, are especially high in vitamins C and A. Raisins and prunes are high in iron. Eating four servings of a variety of fruits and vegetables will help you meet your need for vitamins C and A each day.

Root vegetables also enhance the nutrition of a salad, and you'll find carrots, turnips, jicama, radishes, and beets are excellent choices. All you need to do is add some protein food, such as meat, fish, poultry, beans, eggs, or nuts and seeds, to turn a salad into a whole meal-in-a-dish. Nuts, incidentally, provide excellent protein along with vitamins and minerals to help boost a nutritionally weak salad. They also are high in fat if calories are a concern.

You'll find a salad for every need or whim in these recipes. There are main-dish salads, side-dish salads, sparkling fruit salads, buffet table beauties. And all of them are as low in calories, fats, cholesterol, and salt as we could make them.

Salads require some care to make them as crisp and appealing as possible. Wash greens and shake out any excess moisture to keep them crisp. Wrap well-drained greens in a clean towel or plastic bag and use within a day. It's better to replenish the vegetable bin than risk deterioration of nutrients as well as looks by storing them too long.

Keep salads chilled (not ice cold) until ready to serve. Adding the dressing at the last moment will prevent wilting, unless the recipe specifies earlier use of the dressing.

Vegetable Salads

AVOCADO SALAD

¼ cup Soy Sauce (p. 209)
¼ cup dry white wine
3 avocados
Lettuce leaves
Lemon wedges

Combine Soy Sauce and wine and chill. When ready to serve, cut avocados in half lengthwise and remove pits, but do not peel.

Arrange avocado halves on a bed of lettuce leaves on a platter or on individual plates. Pour about 1½ tablespoons of the chilled soy mixture into each avocado cavity. Garnish with lemon wedges. Makes 6 servings.

Each serving contains about:
195 calories
48 mg sodium
19 g fat
0 mg cholesterol
Exchanges: 4 fat

CALIFORNIA TOSTADA

This handsome meal-in-a-dish, do-it-yourself salad-sandwich borrowed from the Mexican cuisine makes wonderful party food. Stack the toasted tortillas, place the fillings in separate bowls, and allow guests to make their own highrise salads. Just double, triple, or quadruple the recipe according to the size of the crowd.

6 corn tortillas
1¼ cups shredded cooked chicken, pork, or beef
1¼ cups shredded iceberg lettuce
1¼ cups chopped tomatoes
1¼ cups grated low-sodium Cheddar cheese
¾ cup Spanish Sauce (p. 194)
6 tablespoons Guacamole (p. 14, optional)
6 tablespoons low-calorie sour cream
2 tablespoons minced green onion
Cilantro sprigs (fresh coriander)

Place tortillas on an oven rack and bake at 450°F until toasted and crisp. Place each tortilla on a dinner plate. Top each tortilla with about 3 tablespoons *each* chicken, lettuce, tomato, and Cheddar cheese, 2 tablespoons Spanish Sauce, and 1 tablespoon Guacamole. Top each tostada with 1 tablespoon sour cream. Sprinkle with green onion and garnish with cilantro sprigs. Makes 6 servings.

Each tostada with Guacamole contains about:
281 calories

234 mg sodium
12 g fat
59 mg cholesterol
Exchanges: 1 bread, 1 meat, 1 vegetable, 1 fat

CHINESE CHICKEN SALAD

3 chicken breasts (about 1½ pounds boned weight)
½ cup low-sodium Chicken Stock (p. 40)
1 head iceberg lettuce, shredded
4 green onions, sliced
¼ cup chopped cilantro (fresh coriander)
1 (4-ounce) can water chestnuts, thinly sliced
1 stalk celery, thinly sliced
3 radishes, thinly sliced
2 tablespoons sesame seeds, toasted*
Rice Vinegar Dressing (p. 182)

Skin, bone, and split chicken breasts. Place breasts in a skillet with stock, cover, and cook over low heat for 10 to 15 minutes. Remove from stock and let cool. Dice chicken meat and combine with lettuce, onions, cilantro, water chestnuts, celery, radishes, and sesame seeds. Drizzle with Rice Vinegar Dressing and toss to mix well. Makes 6 servings.

*To toast sesame seeds, place in a dry pan over medium heat and heat, stirring, until golden.

Each serving with dressing contains about:
227 calories
108 mg sodium
8 g fat
60 mg cholesterol
Exchanges: 3 meat, 1 vegetable

COLESLAW DE LUXE

¾ cup low-fat plain yogurt
½ cup low-fat vanilla yogurt
2 tablespoons low-sodium, low-calorie mayonnaise
1 tablespoon fresh lemon juice
½ teaspoon celery seeds
1 tablespoon chopped chives
⅛ teaspoon pepper
1 head cabbage, shredded
1 small carrot, grated
1 (4-ounce) can unsweetened crushed
    pineapple, well drained

Mix together yogurts and mayonnaise until smooth. Add lemon juice, celery seeds, chives, and pepper and mix well. Fold in cabbage, carrots, and pineapple until evenly coated. Chill. Makes 12 servings.

Each ½ cup serving contains about:
    40 calories
    20 mg sodium
    3 g fat
    3 mg cholesterol
    Exchanges: 1 vegetable, ½ fat

CUCUMBERS IN YOGURT

2 large cucumbers, peeled
1 cup low-fat plain yogurt
1 tablespoon fresh lemon juice
¼ teaspoon pepper
1 tablespoon *each* chopped parsley and chives or
    green onion tops
¼ teaspoon Worcestershire sauce (optional)
Boston lettuce leaves

Cut cucumbers in half lengthwise and scrape out seeds with a spoon. Cut into thin slices horizontally. Place slices in a tea towel and gently squeeze out excess moisture; set aside.

160   Light Style

Beat yogurt with a wire whisk until smooth. Add lemon juice, pepper, parsley, chives, and Worcestershire sauce. Add cucumber slices and toss to coat well. Chill 1 hour. Serve on a bed of lettuce leaves. Makes 8 servings.

Each ½ cup serving contains about:
25 calories
22 mg sodium
trace fat
trace cholesterol
Exchanges: 1 vegetable

ENDIVE-WATERCRESS SALAD

1 large or 2 small Belgian endives
1 bunch watercress
⅓ cup Lemon Dressing (p. 180)
1 tablespoon chopped pecans
1 tomato, cut in wedges

Cut large endive into eighths and small ones into quarters lengthwise. Immerse in cold water and let soak for 10 minutes. Drain and dry well. Chill 1 hour before using. (Endive should be crisp when ready to use.) Wash, drain, and dry watercress. Wrap in a clean dry cloth and refrigerate until ready to use. Just before serving, combine endive and watercress in a bowl. Add dressing and toss. Sprinkle with pecans and garnish with tomato wedges. Makes 6 servings.

Each 1 cup serving contains about:
42 calories
3 mg sodium
3 g fat
0 mg cholesterol
Exchanges: ½ fat

FABULOUS SALAD

1 bunch spinach
1 small head butter lettuce
1 small head red leaf lettuce
¼ head romaine lettuce
2 tablespoons chopped chives
2 tablespoons chopped parsley
1 teaspoon dried tarragon
2 teaspoons Dijon Mustard (p. 203)
3 tablespoons egg substitute, or 1 egg
Juice of 1 lemon
3 tablespoons vegetable oil
½ cup low-calorie sour cream or low-fat plain yogurt
Dash hot pepper sauce
1 teaspoon fructose
1 cup cooked tiny bay shrimp or small shrimp, deveined
Pepper to taste

Tear spinach and lettuces in bite-size pieces and combine with chives and parsley. Chill. In a small bowl, combine tarragon, mustard, egg substitute or egg, and lemon juice and stir briskly to blend well. Slowly add oil, beating constantly until thickened. Stir in sour cream, hot pepper sauce, and fructose. Add to greens with shrimp and toss to coat well. Sprinkle generously with pepper. Makes 12 servings.

NOTE: If on a low-cholesterol diet, substitute Alaskan king crab for shrimp.

Each 1 cup serving contains about:
73 calories
44 mg sodium
6 g fat
39 mg cholesterol
Exchanges: 1 B vegetable, 1 fat

GINGHAM SALAD

1 cup low-fat cottage cheese
¼ teaspoon celery seeds
3 tablespoons chopped chives
1½ cups coarsely chopped spinach leaves
2 cups shredded red cabbage
6 large lettuce leaves
6 tablespoons Buttermilk-Cucumber
    Dressing (p. 177)

Combine cottage cheese, celery seeds, and chives in a bowl and mix well. Add spinach and cabbage and toss to coat well. For each serving, place a ½-cup serving on a lettuce leaf and top with 1 tablespoon dressing. Makes 6 servings.

Each ½ cup serving contains about:
48 calories
178 mg sodium
trace fat
1 mg cholesterol
Exchanges: ½ meat

MARINATED MUSHROOMS

1 pound large mushrooms, sliced
2 tablespoons chopped parsley
1 teaspoon dried tarragon
¼ cup Lemon Dressing (p. 180)

Combine mushroom slices, parsley, and tarragon in a bowl. Pour dressing over mushroom mixture and toss to coat well. Chill at least 1 hour before serving. Makes 6 servings.

Each ½ cup serving contains about:
31 calories
6 mg sodium
2 g fat
0 mg cholesterol
Exchanges: 1 vegetable, ¼ fat

MEDITERRANEAN SALAD

1 cucumber, sliced
1 bunch radishes, trimmed
1 red bell pepper, cut in strips
1 green bell pepper, cut in strips
3 tomatoes, cut in wedges
½ bunch chicory or curly endive lettuce, shredded
6 green onions, sliced
¼ cup Oregano Dressing (p. 181)
2 tablespoons crumbled feta cheese, or
   low-sodium cheese

Combine cucumber, radishes, peppers, tomatoes, chicory, and onions in a bowl. Drizzle with Oregano Dressing and toss. Sprinkle with feta cheese. Makes 6 servings.
NOTE: Use low-sodium cheese if on a sodium-restricted diet.

Each ½ cup serving with dressing and cheese contains about:
   45 calories
   59 mg sodium
   3 g fat
   4 mg cholesterol
   Exchanges: 1 vegetable, 1 fat

ORANGE-CAULIFLOWER SALAD

3 oranges, peeled and sectioned, or
   2 (10½-ounce) cans unsweetened mandarin
   orange segments, drained
1 medium head cauliflower, separated in flowerets
½ cup chopped green bell pepper
2 cups chopped spinach leaves
¼ cup Orange Blossom Dressing (p. 180)
Lettuce leaves
2 tablespoons slivered almonds

Combine orange segments, cauliflowerets, green pepper, spinach, and Orange Blossom Dressing in a bowl. Toss and place 1 cup salad on lettuce leaf for each serving. Sprinkle with almonds. Makes 6 servings.

Each 1 cup serving contains about:
  55 calories
  26 mg sodium
  1 g fat
  0 mg cholesterol
  Exchanges: 1 fruit

SCANDINAVIAN CUCUMBERS

  2 medium cucumbers, thinly sliced
  1 small onion, thinly sliced
  ½ cup rice or tarragon vinegar
  ½ cup water
  1 tablespoon fructose
  2 sprigs fresh dill, chopped, or
      1 teaspoon dill weed

Combine cucumber and onion slices in a bowl. Combine vinegar, water, and fructose and pour over cucumber mixture. Cover and chill at least 2 hours. Drain, then sprinkle with dill to serve. Makes 6 servings.

Each ½ cup serving contains about:
  21 calories
  4 mg sodium
  0 g fat
  0 mg cholesterol
  Exchanges: 1 vegetable

TOMATO-CAULIFLOWER SALAD

  1 medium head cauliflower, separated in flowerets
  2 tomatoes, cut in wedges
  1 onion, thinly sliced
  3 tablespoons chopped parsley
  ¼ cup Herb Dressing (p. 179)

Cook flowerets in 1 inch boiling water until tender, about 15 minutes; drain. Combine flowerets, tomatoes, onion, parsley, and dressing and marinate 1 hour. Serve at room temperature. Makes 6 servings.

NOTE: If using red onion, do not add it until after the salad has marinated, as the red color will leach out and discolor salad. Add and toss just before serving.

Each ½ cup serving contains about:
45 calories
21 mg sodium
3 g fat
0 mg cholesterol
Exchanges: 1 vegetable, ½ fat

TOMATO-MUSHROOM SALAD

½ pound mushrooms, sliced
2 medium tomatoes, sliced ¼ inch thick
½ cup thinly sliced green onions
2 tablespoons chopped parsley or
   cilantro (fresh coriander)
¼ cup Basil Dressing (p. 177)

Combine mushrooms, tomatoes, onions, and parsley in a bowl. Add Basil Dressing and toss to coat well. Chill at least 1 hour. Makes 6 servings.

Each ½ cup serving with dressing contains about:
46 calories
8 mg sodium
3 g fat
0 mg cholesterol
Exchanges: 1 vegetable, ½ fat

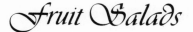

Fruit Salads

AVOCADO-ORANGE SALAD

1 avocado, peeled, pitted,
  and thinly sliced lengthwise
2 oranges or grapefruits,
  peeled and sectioned
1 small head butter or romaine lettuce
⅓ cup Lemon Dressing (p. 180), or
  Oregano Dressing (p. 181)
Fresh mint sprigs or chopped mint

For each serving, arrange 2 avocado slices and 3 citrus slices alternately on a bed of lettuce leaves. Sprinkle with 1 tablespoon dressing of choice and garnish with mint. Makes 6 servings.

Each serving contains about:
112 calories
4 mg sodium
9 g fat
0 mg cholesterol
Exchanges: 1 fruit, 1½ fat

CALIFORNIA SALAD

2 grapefruits, peeled and sectioned
2 oranges, peeled and sectioned, or
    1 (10½-ounce) can unsweetened mandarin
    orange segments, drained
Butter lettuce leaves
⅓ cup Buttermilk-Cucumber Dressing (p. 177)
2 tablespoons slivered almonds, toasted*

For each serving, arrange 3 grapefruit sections and 4 orange segments on a leaf of lettuce. Drizzle with 1 tablespoon Buttermilk-

Cucumber Dressing. Garnish with toasted almonds. Makes 6 servings.

*To toast almonds, place in a dry pan over medium heat and heat, stirring, until golden.

Each 1 cup serving without dressing contains about:
55 calories
5 mg sodium
1 g fat
0 mg cholesterol
Exchanges: 1 fruit

CANTALOUPE CRAB BOATS

3 small cantaloupes
Romaine lettuce leaves
1 cup diced celery
1 pound Alaskan king crab meat, shredded
        (fresh or frozen), or 2 (6½-ounce) cans water-
        packed, unsalted tuna, drained
6 tablespoons Green Goddess Yogurt
        Dressing (p. 179)

Cut cantaloupes in half crosswise. Scoop out and discard seeds. Using a serrated flexible knife, cut out flesh, leaving shells intact. Dice cantaloupe flesh. Line each cantaloupe shell with lettuce leaves. Combine diced cantaloupe, celery, and crab meat and pile into melon shells. Cover and chill at least 20 minutes. Place each shell on a bed of lettuce leaves on a plate. Top each salad with 1 tablespoon Green Goddess Yogurt Dressing. Makes 6 servings.

NOTE: Canned crab has a high salt content. We suggest that those watching their salt intake use only fresh or frozen Alaskan king crab meat.

Each serving with dressing contains about:
145 calories
42 mg sodium (content unavailable for crab)
2 g fat
77 mg cholesterol
Exchanges: 2½ meat, 1 fruit

CHICKEN-STUFFED PAPAYA

3 chicken breasts (about 1½ pounds boned weight)
1 cup low-sodium Chicken Stock, (p. 40)
⅓ cup low-sodium, low-calorie mayonnaise
⅓ cup low-fat plain yogurt
½ teaspoon dry mustard
1 tablespoon fresh lime juice
½ cup chopped celery
2 tablespoons chopped green onion
2 tablespoons chopped chives
½ teaspoon ground ginger or curry powder
Pepper to taste
3 papayas
Lettuce leaves
2 tablespoons slivered almonds, toasted*
Watercress or parsley sprigs or lime slices (optional)

Skin, bone, and split chicken breasts. Place chicken in a skillet and add stock. Cover and simmer 10 to 15 minutes, or until chicken is tender. Drain, cool, and cube chicken. Combine mayonnaise, yogurt, mustard, lime juice, celery, onion, chives, ginger, and pepper and blend well. Add cubed chicken and toss to coat well. Chill.

Peel and halve papayas. Scoop out and discard seeds. Arrange each papaya half on a serving plate lined with lettuce leaves. Pile chicken salad in papaya cavities and sprinkle with almonds. Garnish with watercress sprigs, if desired. Makes 6 servings.

*To toast almonds, place in a dry pan over medium heat and heat, stirring, until golden.

Each serving contains about:
225 calories
77 mg sodium
8 g fat
61 mg cholesterol
Exchanges: 3 meat, 1 fruit

BLOSSOM PEACH SALAD

⅓ cup Cream Cheese (p. 208)
2 tablespoons chopped pecans
6 ripe peaches
Fresh lemon juice
Watercress sprigs
2 tablespoons Orange Blossom
    Dressing (p. 180)
Mint leaves

Divide cheese into 6 equal portions. Form each portion into a ball, then roll in chopped nuts. Peel and pit peaches and cut in half if using fresh peaches. Place a ball of cheese between 2 peach halves and press back into shape of peach. Brush with lemon juice to prevent discoloration. (Omit this step if using canned peaches.) Chill in a covered container until ready to use. Place each stuffed peach on a bed of watercress. Drizzle each peach with 1 teaspoon Orange Blossom Dressing and garnish with mint leaves. Makes 6 servings.

NOTE: Any fresh fruit or fruit canned in water may be substituted for the peaches.

Each serving without dressing contains about:
78 calories
32 mg sodium
3 g fat
3 mg cholesterol
Exchanges: 1 fruit, ½ fat

WALDORF SALAD

A low-caloried twist to a favorite classic salad.

Juice of 1 lemon
3 red Delicious apples, diced
1 cup diced celery
¼ cup raisins
⅓ cup pecans or walnuts, chopped
¾ cup low-fat vanilla yogurt
Lettuce leaves

Sprinkle lemon juice over diced apples to prevent discoloration. Combine apples, celery, raisins, pecans, and yogurt in a bowl. Toss to coat well. Arrange on a bed of lettuce. Makes 12 servings.

Each ½ cup serving contains about:
  44 calories
  19 mg sodium
  3 g fat
  trace cholesterol
  Exchanges: ½ fat, 1 fruit

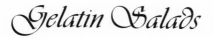

Gelatin Salads

AUTUMN SALAD

2 (⅝-ounce) packages regular or low-calorie
    lime-flavored gelatin
2 cups boiling water
1 (8-ounce) can unsweetened crushed pineapple
1 cup grated carrots
¼ cup chopped walnuts
¼ cup low-sodium, low-calorie mayonnaise

Dissolve gelatin in boiling water. Drain pineapple, reserving juice. Combine reserved juice and enough cold water to make 1 cup. Stir into gelatin mixture and chill until syrupy. Fold in drained pineapple, carrots, and walnuts and turn into an 8-inch square pan. Chill until firm. Cut into squares to serve. Top each serving with 1 teaspoon mayonnaise. Makes 12 servings.

Each serving (2⅔-by-2⅔ inch) contains about:
  121 calories (57 calories if using low-calorie gelatin)
  74 mg sodium (28 mg sodium if using low-calorie gelatin)
  3 g fat
  0 mg cholesterol
  Exchanges: 1 bread, ½ fruit, ½ fat (½ fruit, ½ fat if using
    low-calorie gelatin)

SUNSHINE SALAD

2 (⅝-ounce) packages regular or low-calorie
    lemon-flavored gelatin
2 cups boiling water
1 (8-ounce) can unsweetened mandarin
    orange sections
1 (8-ounce) can unsweetened crushed pineapple
1 (4-ounce) can unsweetened grapefruit sections
½ cup Heavenly Whipped Topping (p. 205)
2 tablespoons toasted unsweetened
    shredded coconut

Dissolve gelatin in boiling water. Drain juice from cans of orange, pineapple and grapefruit, reserving 2 cups juice. Stir reserved juice into gelatin mixture. Chill until syrupy. Fold in well-drained fruit. Turn into an 8-inch square pan and chill until firm. Spread Heavenly Whipped Topping over gelatin. Sprinkle with toasted coconut. Cut into squares to serve. Makes 9 servings.

    Each serving (2⅔-by-2⅔ inches) contains about:
      106 calories (43 calories if using low-calorie gelatin)
      71 mg sodium (6 mg sodium if using low-calorie gelatin)
      trace fat
      0 mg cholesterol
      Exchanges: 1 bread, 1 fruit (1 fruit if using low-calorie gelatin)

HOLIDAY SALAD

2 (⅝-ounce) packages regular or low-calorie
    strawberry-flavored gelatin
1 quart boiling water
1 basket strawberries, hulled and sliced, or
    1 (10-ounce) package frozen, unsweetened
    strawberries, thawed
1 (20-ounce) can unsweetened pineapple
    chunks, drained
1 cup Cream Cheese (p. 208)
1 cup low-fat strawberry or vanilla yogurt
1 cup Heavenly Whipped Topping (p. 205)

Dissolve gelatin in boiling water. Chill until syrupy. Fold in strawberries and pineapple. Pour half the mixture into a 1½-quart mold and chill until just firm. Spread Cream Cheese evenly over set gelatin, then spread strawberry yogurt over cream cheese. Pour remaining gelatin mixture over yogurt. Chill at least 24 hours. Unmold onto serving plate. Serve with Heavenly Whipped Topping. Makes 12 servings.

Each ½ cup serving with topping contains about:
138 calories (75 calories if using low-calorie gelatin)
88 mg sodium (50 mg sodium if using low-calorie gelatin)
trace fat
5 mg cholesterol
Exchanges: 1 bread, 1 fruit, ¼ milk (1 fruit, ¼ milk if using low-calorie gelatin)

Salad Dressings

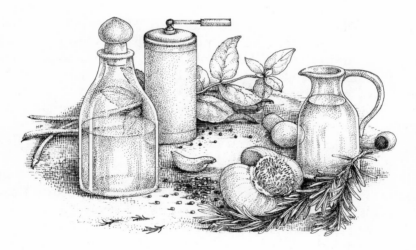

Consider this: 1 tablespoon of regular salad dressing contains about 100 calories and 180 mg sodium. *Light Style* dressings contain an average of 30 calories per tablespoon and 17 mg sodium, which makes the case for preparing your own low-calorie, low-sodium, low-fat salad dressings all that much more appealing. And at a fraction of the cost of the commercial brands, you can't go wrong!

You will learn, by using these recipes, how to modify your own dressing concoctions. To lower cholesterol, for instance, we use safflower oil. Fructose is used in place of sugar to reduce total calories. Cream dressings make use of low-fat cottage cheese, buttermilk (naturally low in fat but higher in sodium than whole milk), low-fat yogurt, and evaporated nonfat milk, plus low-calorie mayonnaise, which you can buy as "imitation" mayonnaise or make.

The missing salt in the recipes is compensated for in the use of herbs, fruit juices, and flavored vinegars. Fresh herbs are more effective flavor-enhancers than dried.

If you use vinegar-based dressings frequently, it might be a good idea to prepare several batches and store them in jars with tight-fitting lids for up to a month. Creamy dressings should be stored in the refrigerator no longer than a week. Always shake or mix dressings until smooth and well reconstituted before using.

BASIL DRESSING

¼ cup safflower oil
3 tablespoons wine vinegar or rice vinegar, or
    fresh lemon juice
¼ cup water
2 tablespoons minced fresh basil, or
    1½ teaspoons dried basil
1 teaspoon finely chopped garlic
1½ teaspoons fructose
Pepper to taste

Combine oil, vinegar, water, basil, garlic, fructose, and pepper to taste in blender container. Blend until smooth. Makes ¾ cup.

Each 1 tablespoon serving contains about:
    41 calories
    0 mg sodium
    4 g fat
    0 mg cholesterol
    Exchanges: 1 fat

BUTTERMILK-CUCUMBER DRESSING

¼ cup buttermilk
2¼ tablespoons low-fat cottage cheese
1½ tablespoons fresh lemon juice
1 teaspoon dill weed, or
    1 tablespoon chopped fresh dill
1 clove garlic, minced
Pepper to taste
½ cucumber, peeled and diced
⅓ cup diced red bell pepper or
    sliced radishes (optional)

Mix together buttermilk, cottage cheese, lemon juice, dill, garlic, and pepper. Stir in cucumber and red pepper. Chill. Makes about ¾ cup.

Each 2-tablespoon serving contains about:
15 calories
27 mg sodium
trace fat
1 mg cholesterol
Exchanges: negligible

CREAMY GARLIC DRESSING

1¼ cups low-fat plain yogurt
½ cup nonfat milk or evaporated nonfat milk
4 cloves garlic, minced
1 teaspoon dried basil, or
   1 tablespoon chopped fresh basil
1 teaspoon dried oregano, or
   1 tablespoon chopped fresh oregano
1 teaspoon dried rosemary, or
   1 tablespoon chopped fresh rosemary
1 teaspoon dried sage, or
   1 tablespoon chopped fresh sage
1 teaspoon dill weed, or
   1 tablespoon chopped fresh dill

Combine yogurt, milk, garlic, basil, oregano, rosemary, sage, and dill in blender container and blend until smooth. Makes about 1¾ cups.

Each 2 tablespoon serving contains about:
14 calories
14 mg sodium
trace fat
trace cholesterol
Exchanges: negligible

GREEN GODDESS YOGURT DRESSING

2 tablespoons white wine vinegar or
    rice vinegar
¾ teaspoon dried tarragon, or
    1 tablespoon chopped fresh tarragon
1½ tablespoons chopped green onion or chives
3 tablespoons minced parsley
1 teaspoon fructose
¾ cup low-fat plain yogurt
¼ cup low-sodium, low-calorie mayonnaise

Combine vinegar, tarragon, onion, parsley, fructose, yogurt, and
mayonnaise in a blender container. Blend until smooth and very
green, 2 to 3 minutes. Makes about 1½ cups.

Each 1 tablespoon serving contains about:
    13 calories
    4 mg sodium
    1 g fat
    trace cholesterol
    Exchanges: negligible

HERB DRESSING

6 tablespoons safflower oil
2 teaspoons chopped parsley
2 teaspoons chopped chives
2 teaspoons dried chervil, or
    2 tablespoons chopped fresh chervil
Pepper to taste
½ cup rice vinegar
2 tablespoons water
3 cloves garlic, minced
2 teaspoons dry mustard

Combine oil, parsley, chives, chervil, pepper, vinegar, water, garlic,
and dry mustard in a blender container. Blend well. Makes 1 cup.

Each 1 tablespoon serving contains about:
  46 calories
  16 mg sodium
  5 g fat
  0 mg cholesterol
  Exchanges: 1 fat

LEMON DRESSING

  ¼ cup fresh lemon juice
  2 tablespoons water
  1 teaspoon Dijon Mustard (p. 203)
  Pinch cayenne pepper
  2 tablespoons olive oil or vegetable oil
  ½ teaspoon dried chervil, or
      1½ teaspoons chopped fresh chervil
  ½ teaspoon dried tarragon, or
      1½ teaspoons chopped fresh tarragon
  2 tablespoons chopped pecans (optional)

Combine lemon juice, water, mustard and pepper in a blender container and blend well. Add oil, chervil, and tarragon and blend to a smooth sauce. Mix in nuts, if desired. Makes ½ cup.

  Each 1 tablespoon serving without pecans contains about:
    37 calories
    1 mg sodium
    3 g fat
    0 mg cholesterol
    Exchanges: ½ fat

ORANGE BLOSSOM DRESSING

  1 cup low-fat plain yogurt
  ½ cup evaporated nonfat milk
  1 (6-ounce) can frozen unsweetened
      orange juice concentrate, thawed

Combine yogurt, milk, and orange juice in a blender container and blend well. Makes 2½ cups.

Each 1 tablespoon serving contains about:
15 calories
5 mg sodium
trace fat
trace cholesterol
Exchanges: ½ fruit

OREGANO DRESSING

3 tablespoons red wine vinegar or rice vinegar
1 tablespoon water
1 tablespoon fresh lemon juice
3 tablespoons olive oil
2 tablespoons minced parsley
¾ teaspoon dried oregano, or
   1 tablespoon chopped fresh oregano
Pepper to taste

Combine vinegar, water, lemon juice, oil, parsley, oregano, and pepper in a blender container and blend thoroughly. Let stand at least 1 hour before using to allow flavors to blend. Makes ½ cup.

Each 1 tablespoon serving contains about:
46 calories
trace sodium
5 g fat
0 mg cholesterol
Exchanges: 1 fat

RICE VINEGAR DRESSING

The rice vinegar provides a sweet delicate flavor.

    ¼ cup corn oil
    3 tablespoons rice vinegar
    1 teaspoon fructose
    1 tablespoon water
    Pepper to taste

Combine oil, vinegar, fructose, water, and pepper in a small jar and shake until well blended. Makes ½ cup.

    Each 1 tablespoon serving contains about:
        62 calories
        trace sodium
        7 g fat
        0 mg cholesterol
        Exchanges: 1 fat

VINAIGRETTE

        3 tablespoons safflower oil
    1½ teaspoons olive oil
        3 tablespoons plus 1 teaspoon fresh lemon juice
        1 tablespoon water
    ½ teaspoon Dijon Mustard (p. 203)
        Pepper to taste
    ¼ teaspoon capers, minced*
    ⅛ teaspoon dill weed, or
        ½ teaspoon chopped fresh dill
    ½ teaspoon dried chervil, or
        1½ teaspoons chopped fresh chervil (optional)
        1 teaspoon *each* chopped parsley and chives
        1 teaspoon fructose

In a small bowl, combine safflower oil, olive oil, lemon juice, water, mustard, pepper, capers, dill, chervil, parsley, chives, and fructose. Blend with a wire whisk until well blended. Chill. Makes about ½ cup.

182   Light Style

*One teaspoon of capers contains 100 milligrams sodium.

Each 1 tablespoon serving contains about:
59 calories
13 mg sodium
6 g fat
0 mg cholesterol
Exchanges: 1 fat

LOW-CALORIE RUSSIAN DRESSING

2 teaspoons unflavored gelatin
¼ cup rice vinegar
¼ cup boiling water
½ cup Catsup (p. 203)
1½ teaspoons Worcestershire sauce
2 tablespoons finely minced onion
Pepper to taste
2 tablespoons safflower oil

Soften gelatin in 2 tablespoons of the rice vinegar. Dissolve gelatin mixture in boiling water. Cool. Stir in remaining rice vinegar, Catsup, Worcestershire sauce, onion, pepper, and oil. Beat well with a wire whisk. Chill. Before serving, shake well or beat with wire whisk. Makes about 1¼ cups.

Each 1 tablespoon serving contains about:
22 calories
7 mg sodium
1 g fat
0 mg cholesterol
Exchanges: negligible

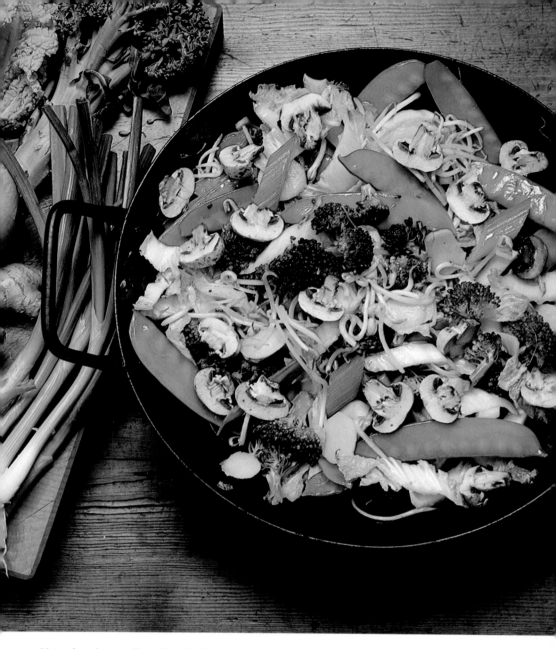

Using broth as well as oil is the low-calorie, low-fat approach to these Chinese Stir-Fry Vegetables. Broccoli, cauliflower, celery, snow peas, Chinese cabbage, mushrooms, bamboo shoots, bean sprouts, and water chestnuts are quickly stir-fried to bring out full flavor, beautiful color, and crisp texture. Quick cooking helps preserve nutrients, too.

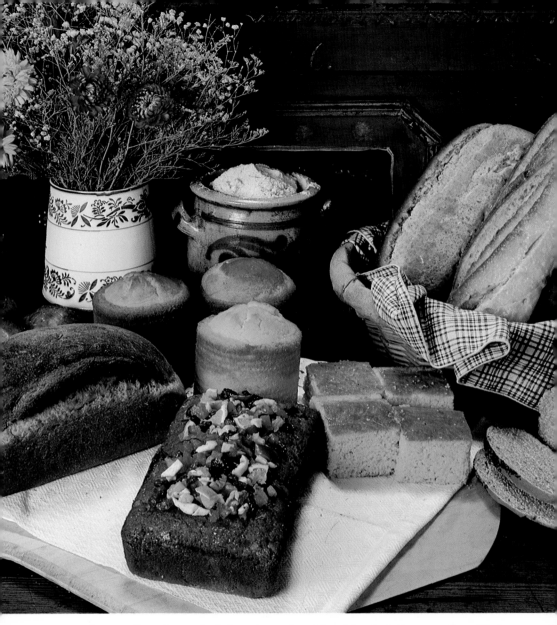

Low-sodium, low-calorie breads, made with unbleached flour, nonfat milk, low-calorie margarine, and fructose, are, from left: big, ballooning Popovers, made with nonfat milk and egg substitute; a poppyseed-covered loaf of Ramona's Whole Wheat Bread; Corn Bread baked in coffee cans; Holiday Bread, a quick bread topped with nuts, apple, orange peel, and currants; Corn Bread baked in a pan and cut into squares; French Bread; and Ramona's Whole Wheat Bread, sliced.

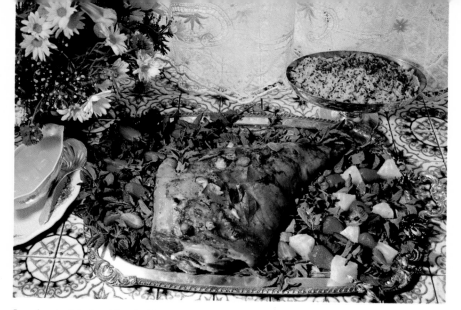

Lamb studded with shallots and garlic, rubbed generously with herbs (and trimmed of all excess fat), is roasted to serve with Pineapple Sauce and naturally low-calorie strawberries and fresh pineapple on skewers. Wild Rice Casserole is a fitting companion.

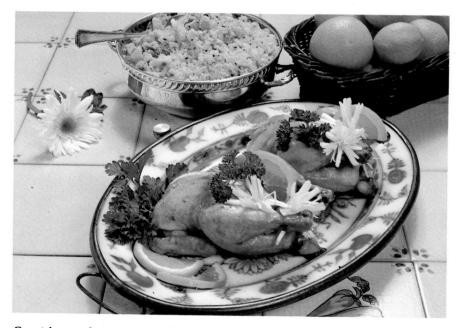

Cornish game hens are garnished with orange slices and green onion tops, slivered and fanned to form blossoms. The Herb Corn Bread Stuffing is baked separately to reduce fat.

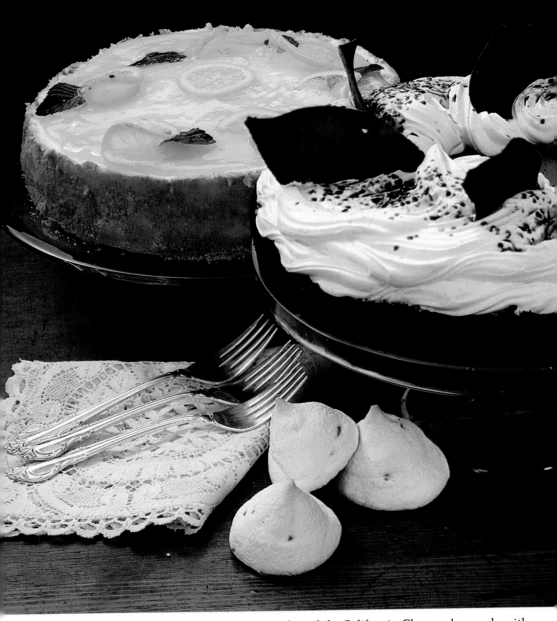

A trio of low-calorie desserts are, from left: California Cheesecake, made with naturally low-calorie ricotta cheese and yogurt; Chocolate Mousse Pie, made with real chocolate, egg whites, and fructose, and topped with an 8-calorie-per-table-spoon gelatin-based whipped topping; and Snow Drop Cookies, made with frothy egg whites, sweetened with fructose, and studded with chocolate, at a mere 30 calories per cookie.

Sauces, Condiments, and Specialty Recipes

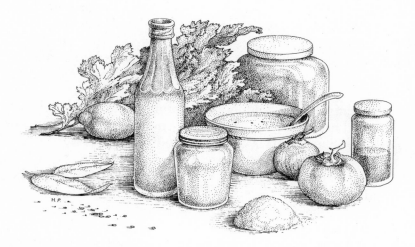

$\mathcal{A}$ low-sodium catsup? Low-calorie French sauces you would swear were riddled with calories but aren't? A hollandaise without eggs? A Madeira sauce without fat?

What a blessing to be able to control the salt, fat, sugar, eggs, and calories in your sauces and condiments. And they're all yours for the making at the lowest cost and highest quality possible.

Condiments rarely add nutritional value to foods, but they are important flavoring agents. For the *Light Style* cook who is concerned about salt and fat content of foods, they can be a preventive health tool.

Our sauces make use of low-calorie margarine to reduce both calories and cholesterol. Arrowroot and cornstarch provide lower calories than flour because you need less of them to thicken foods. Calorie-lowering fructose is used in place of sugar because less is needed for sweetening food. Low-sodium canned tomatoes are allowed to co-exist with fresh ones for convenience sake. Wine is a reliable flavor enhancer, especially in sauces. For sauces using cheese, we employ the low-sodium brands found commercially. Unsweetened fruit juices and fruit also contribute flavor along with fewer calories. Sauces calling for dairy products almost always make use of nonfat types. Low-sodium stocks you make yourself using our recipes or you buy commercially help reduce total sodium intake. Homemade stocks add extra flavor, too.

Condiments such as catsup, mustard, Herb Blend, and Soy Sauce can be stored up to one month with no worry of spoilage, if you observe good rules of food safety. Store them in the refrigerator in containers with tight-fitting lids. Sauces should be stored no longer than up to a week in the refrigerator for safety's sake.

You might also keep in mind that condiments and unusual sauces make charming gifts when packed in pretty jars with labels. You might even add the recipe for an appreciative friend.

BECHAMEL SAUCE
White Sauce

2 tablespoons low-calorie margarine
2 tablespoons flour
½ cup nonfat milk
½ cup evaporated nonfat milk
Pinch white pepper

Melt margarine in a saucepan. Stir in flour until smooth. Gradually stir in milks. Continue to cook and stir until sauce comes to a boil. Reduce heat and simmer 2 to 3 minutes, stirring constantly, until sauce is thickened and smooth. Season with pepper. Makes about 1¼ cups.

   Each 1 tablespoon serving contains about:
   21 calories
   23 mg sodium
   0 g fat
   trace cholesterol
   Exchanges: negligible

BLENDER BEARNAISE

Light Style Béarnaise has half the calories and fat of the classic version.

  2 tablespoons *each* white wine vinegar and
      dry white wine
1½ teaspoons minced shallots or green onion
  ¼ teaspoon dried tarragon, or
      ¾ teaspoon chopped fresh tarragon
  Dash paprika
  Dash cayenne pepper
  6 tablespoons egg substitute, or 2 egg yolks
  2 tablespoons low-calorie margarine, melted
  1 tablespoon fresh lemon juice

Combine vinegar, wine, shallots, tarragon, paprika, and cayenne pepper in a small saucepan and bring to a boil. Boil until liquid has reduced to about 1 tablespoon. Pour into a blender container and let cool. Add egg substitute or yolks to blender container and blend until smooth. With the blender motor running at low speed, add the melted margarine in a fine steady stream. Pour sauce into top of a double boiler placed over simmering water. Cook and stir until sauce thickens, about 1 minute. Remove from heat. Makes ½ cup.

NOTE: To reheat Béarnaise, place it in the top pan of a double boiler placed over hot water and stir just until sauce is warm and reconstituted.

  Each 2 tablespoon serving contains about:
  40 calories
  80 mg sodium
  6 g fat
  0 mg cholesterol
  Exchanges: 1 fat

CHICKEN OR TURKEY GRAVY

3 tablespoons low-calorie margarine
1 clove garlic, minced
2 tablespoons arrowroot
1½ cups low-sodium Chicken or
    Turkey Stock (p. 40), heated
1 bay leaf
¼ cup white wine

Melt margarine in a saucepan. Add garlic and cook about 30 seconds. Stir in arrowroot until smooth. Add stock, bay leaf, and wine and cook and stir until sauce thickens, about 5 minutes. Remove bay leaf. Serve with meat or poultry. Makes about 2 cups.

Each 3 tablespoon serving contains about:
27 calories
36 mg sodium
2 g fat
trace cholesterol
Exchanges: ¼ fat

DRAWN MARGARINE

Margarine does not contain milk solids, so it's unnecessary to melt down milky residue as you would for butter.

6 tablespoons low-calorie margarine
4½ teaspoons fresh lemon juice or white vinegar
1 teaspoon chopped capers
1 tablespoon finely chopped parsley
2 teaspoons finely chopped shallots

Melt margarine in a small saucepan over low heat. Stir in lemon juice, capers, parsley, and shallots all at once. Makes about ½ cup.

Each 1 tablespoon serving contains about:
41 calories

87 mg sodium
4 g fat
0 mg cholesterol
Exchanges: 1 fat

FRENCH PROVINCIAL SAUCE
Brown Sauce

This is the *Light Style* version of the French classic brown sauce used as a base for many sauces added to meat, fish, or fowl.

  2 teaspoons low-sodium tomato purée
  2 teaspoons fructose
  ⅛ teaspoon maple extract
  2 cups low-sodium Beef Stock (p. 39)
  ½ cup plus 1 tablespoon dry red wine
  Bouquet Garni (p. 202)
  ¼ cup chopped onion
1½ tablespoons arrowroot

Combine tomato purée, fructose, maple extract, beef stock, ½ cup of the wine, Bouquet Garni, and onion in a saucepan. Simmer, covered, for 45 minutes. Strain broth through a fine sieve or cheesecloth to measure about 1½ cups. Return broth to the saucepan. Dissolve arrowroot in remaining 1 tablespoon wine. Mix arrowroot mixture into broth with a wire whisk. Place over low heat and simmer, stirring until sauce thickens, about 5 minutes.

Use as much sauce as is needed for one meal and refrigerate remainder in a tightly covered jar for up to 2 days, or freeze in a plastic container leaving 1-inch head space for expansion during freezing for up to 1 month. Makes about 1½ cups.

  Each 1 tablespoon serving contains about:
    11 calories
    1 mg sodium
    trace fat
    trace cholesterol
    Exchanges: negligible

HOLLANDAISE SAUCE

5 tablespoons egg substitute, or 2 egg yolks
Dash *each* paprika and cayenne pepper
1 tablespoon fresh lemon juice
½ teaspoon white wine vinegar
3 tablespoons low-calorie margarine

Combine egg substitute or egg yolks, paprika, cayenne pepper, lemon juice, and vinegar in a blender container and blend at medium speed until smooth. Melt 2 tablespoons of the margarine. With blender motor running at low speed, add margarine in a fine steady stream. Pour sauce into top of a double boiler and place over hot, not boiling, water. Cook, stirring with a wire whisk, until sauce is thickened to the consistency of heavy cream. Beat in remaining 1 tablespoon margarine until well blended. Remove sauce from heat. If not serving immediately, sauce can be reheated by placing over hot water and stirring until warmed. Makes about ½ cup.

Each 1 tablespoon serving contains about:
31 calories
63 mg sodium
4 g fat
0 mg cholesterol
Exchanges: 1 fat

MORNAY SAUCE

1½ tablespoons low-calorie margarine
1 tablespoon arrowroot
1 cup evaporated nonfat milk
Dash ground nutmeg
Dash white pepper
1 tablespoon dry sherry
⅓ cup grated low-sodium Gouda or Cheddar cheese

Melt margarine in a saucepan. Blend in arrowroot until smooth. Add milk all at once. Cook and stir until thickened and bubbly. Add nutmeg and pepper and stir in sherry. Mix in cheese and heat, stirring, until cheese is melted. Makes about 1¼ cups.

Each 2 tablespoon serving contains about:
35 calories
26 mg sodium
1 g fat
3 mg cholesterol
Exchanges: ¼ milk

ITALIAN MEAT SAUCE

Use Italian plum tomatoes when in season for best flavor and texture.

 2 pounds ground beef sirloin
 2 large onions, chopped
 3 cloves garlic, minced
10 Italian plum tomatoes, peeled and diced, or
   1 (20-ounce) can low-sodium tomatoes, diced
 1 (16-ounce) can low-sodium tomato juice
 1 tablespoon dried oregano, or
   3 tablespoons chopped fresh oregano
 1 teaspoon dried thyme, or
   1 tablespoon chopped fresh thyme
½ teaspoon dried marjoram, or
   1½ teaspoons chopped fresh marjoram
 2 teaspoons fennel seeds
 1 teaspoon dried basil, or
   1 tablespoon chopped fresh basil
 1 bay leaf
¾ cup chopped parsley
½ teaspoon pepper
½ cup dry red wine (preferably Chianti)

Combine meat, onions, and half the garlic in a large saucepan. Sauté until onions are tender and meat is crumbly. Add tomatoes, tomato juice, remaining garlic, oregano, thyme, marjoram, fennel, basil, bay leaf, parsley, and pepper. Bring to a boil, reduce heat, partially cover, and simmer 2 hours, stirring occasionally. Add wine and simmer 30 minutes longer, stirring occasionally. Remove bay leaf. Makes about 6½ cups.

NOTE: It is necessary to peel the tomatoes to make a thick sauce.

Each ¼ cup serving contains about:
   81 calories
   24 mg sodium
   1 g fat
   30 mg cholesterol
   Exchanges: 1 meat, ½ B vegetable.

ITALIAN TOMATO SAUCE

10 ripe Italian plum tomatoes, peeled and diced, or
      1 (20-ounce) can low-sodium tomatoes with their juice
  2 tablespoons chopped fresh oregano, or
      2 teaspoons dried oregano
½ teaspoon dried thyme, or
      1½ tablespoons chopped fresh thyme
½ teaspoon dried marjoram, or
      1½ teaspoons chopped fresh marjoram
  1 teaspoon fennel seeds
  1 bay leaf
½ large onion, minced
  4 cloves garlic, minced
½ teaspoon white pepper
½ cup dry red wine (preferably Chianti)
¼ cup chopped parsley

In a large saucepan, combine tomatoes, oregano, thyme, marjoram, fennel seeds, bay leaf, onion, garlic, and pepper. Bring to a boil, reduce heat, and simmer, uncovered, for 1 hour, stirring occasionally. Add wine and parsley and simmer 30 minutes. Remove bay leaf. Makes about 5 cups.

Each ¼ cup serving contains about:
   22 calories
   4 mg sodium
   0 g fat
   0 mg cholesterol
   Exchanges: ½ vegetable

MARINARA SAUCE

1 tablespoon olive oil
½ cup finely chopped onion
1½ cups peeled and coarsely chopped fresh tomatoes
1 cup low-sodium canned tomatoes with their liquid
2 teaspoons dried basil, or
    2 tablespoons chopped fresh basil
1 teaspoon fructose
Pepper to taste

Heat oil in a saucepan and add onion. Sauté until golden and tender, about 1 minute. Add fresh and canned tomatoes, basil, fructose, and pepper. Simmer, partially covered, over very low heat for 40 minutes, stirring occasionally. Place cooked tomato mixture in a blender container and purée. Reheat to serve. Makes 2 cups.

Each ¼ cup serving contains about:
35 calories
5 mg sodium
trace fat
0 mg cholesterol
Exchanges: 1 vegetable

SPANISH SAUCE

½ teaspoon olive oil
1 tablespoon low-calorie margarine
1 teaspoon minced garlic
1½ green bell peppers, sliced
1½ medium onions, sliced lengthwise,
    then slices halved crosswise
3 large tomatoes, diced
¼ cup low-sodium tomato juice
1½ cups low-sodium tomato purée*
1 teaspoon dried oregano, or
    1 tablespoon chopped fresh oregano
2 dashes ground cumin

Heat oil and margarine in a skillet and add garlic, green peppers, and onions. Sauté until tender, about 5 to 6 minutes. Add tomatoes, tomato juice, tomato purée, oregano, and cumin to the onion mixture. Simmer, uncovered, for 30 minutes, stirring occasionally. Serve as topping for omelets, fish, chicken, or tacos. Makes 3 cups.

*To make your own low-sodium tomato purée, place fresh peeled tomatoes or low-sodium canned tomatoes in a blender container and blend until smooth.

Each ¼ cup serving contains about:
    35 calories
    16 mg sodium
    trace fat
    0 mg cholesterol
    Exchanges: 1 vegetable

MADEIRA SAUCE

Truffles add an authentic touch to this classic meat sauce, but mushrooms will do, too.

    4½ teaspoons low-calorie margarine
    2 tablespoons minced shallots, or
        2 tablespoons minced onion
    2 cloves garlic, minced
    ½ cup sliced mushrooms, or
        2 tablespoons chopped truffles
    1 cup low-sodium Beef Stock (p. 39)
    ¼ cup Madeira or dry sherry
    1 tablespoon chopped fresh basil, or
        1 teaspoon dried basil
    1 bay leaf
    2½ teaspoons arrowroot
    1 teaspoon water
    Pepper to taste

Melt margarine in a skillet. Add shallots, garlic, and mushrooms and sauté until mushrooms are tender but not brown. Add stock, wine, basil, and bay leaf. Dissolve arrowroot in water and stir into wine mixture with a wire whisk. Cook, stirring, until sauce thickens, about 15 minutes. Remove bay leaf. Season to taste with pepper. Makes about 1¼ cups.

Each 2 tablespoon serving contains about:
25 calories
32 mg sodium
trace fat
trace cholesterol
Exchanges: negligible

SAUCE ABEL

2 tablespoons low-calorie margarine
2 cloves garlic, minced
2 tablespoons arrowroot
1 tablespoon water
1 cup low-sodium Chicken Stock (p. 40) or
    Beef Stock (p. 39), heated
1 cup nonfat milk, heated
1 bay leaf
2 tablespoons dry Sherry (optional)

Melt margarine in a saucepan. Add garlic and cook 15 seconds. Dissolve arrowroot in water and stir into margarine until smooth with a wire whisk. Gradually add stock, milk, and bay leaf and cook and stir until sauce thickens. Remove bay leaf and stir in Sherry, if desired. Makes 2½ cups.

Each ¼ cup serving contains about:
36 calories
44 mg sodium
1 g fat
1 mg cholesterol
Exchanges: negligible

SAUCE VELOUTE

This "neo" classic sauce goes well with fish or shellfish.

2 tablespoons low-calorie margarine
4 shallots, minced
2 tablespoons arrowroot
½ cup plus 1 tablespoon evaporated nonfat milk
1 cup Fish Stock (p. 41)
Pinch *each* white pepper and cayenne pepper

Melt margarine in a saucepan. Add shallots and sauté until tender. Blend together arrowroot and 1 tablespoon of the milk and stir into margarine mixture until smooth. Gradually add stock, the remaining milk, and the white and cayenne peppers. Cook and stir until sauce is smooth and thickened. Makes about 1½ cups.

Each 2 tablespoon serving contains about:
24 calories
16 mg sodium
1 g fat
trace cholesterol
Exchanges: negligible

PINEAPPLE SAUCE

A versatile sauce for both meat and dessert.

¾ cup unsweetened pineapple juice
1 tablespoon fructose
2 teaspoons arrowroot
1 cup canned water-packed, drained
    pineapple chunks

Combine pineapple juice and fructose in a saucepan. Dissolve arrowroot in 1 tablespoon of the pineapple juice mixture and return to pan. Place over medium heat and cook and stir until thickened. Stir in pineapple chunks. Serve with lamb, ham, or ice cream. Makes 1½ cups.

Each 2 tablespoon serving contains about:
22 calories
trace mg sodium
0 g fat
0 mg cholesterol
Exchanges: ½ fruit

TARRAGON SAUCE

1 tablespoon low-calorie margarine
1 tablespoon arrowroot
1 tablespoon water
½ cup low-sodium Chicken Stock (p. 40)
½ cup evaporated nonfat milk
¼ cup dry white wine
½ teaspoon dried tarragon, or
    2 sprigs fresh tarragon, minced
1 clove garlic, minced
Pepper to taste

Melt margarine in a saucepan over medium heat. Dissolve arrowroot in water and stir into margarine until smooth. Gradually add stock, stirring constantly. Continue to cook and stir until smooth and thickened, about 4 minutes. Add milk, wine, tarragon, garlic, and pepper to saucepan and mix well. Continue to cook and stir until smooth. Serve with chicken or other poultry. Makes about 1¼ cups.

Each ¼ cup serving contains about:
56 calories
40 mg sodium
trace fat
trace cholesterol
Exchanges: ½ bread

Sauces, Cold

APPLESAUCE

8 tart green apples, cored, peeled, and sliced
4 red Delicious apples, cored, peeled, and sliced
1½ cups unsweetened apple juice
½ cup water
2 teaspoons ground cinnamon
¼ teaspoon ground nutmeg

Combine apples, apple juice, water, cinnamon, and nutmeg in a large saucepan. Bring to a boil, reduce heat, cover, and simmer until apples are very soft about 45 minutes. Drain off liquid and discard. Mash apples with a fork and return to saucepan. Cook, covered, over very low heat until excess moisture is absorbed and applesauce is light. Let cool and chill. Applesauce may be stored in a covered plastic container in the refrigerator for up to 2 weeks. Makes 2 quarts.

Each ½ cup serving contains about:
70 calories
2 mg sodium
0 g fat
0 mg cholesterol
Exchanges: 1 fruit

CRANBERRY SAUCE

1 cup peeled and chopped apples
1 pound fresh cranberries (4 cups), or
    1 (10-ounce) package frozen cranberries, thawed
1 cup hot water
¼ teaspoon baking soda
1½ teaspoons low-calorie cherry-flavored gelatin

Place apples and cranberries in a 2-quart saucepan. Add water, bring to a boil, and cook until berries pop. Reduce heat and stir in baking soda. Remove from heat. Skim foam from berries and drain, reserving liquid. Dissolve gelatin into hot berry liquid. Chill until syrupy. Fold in berries and spoon into jars with tight-fitting lids. Chill. For the best flavor, prepare the sauce a few days before serving. Makes about 3 cups.

Each 2 tablespoon serving contains about:
19 calories
10 mg sodium
0 g fat
0 mg cholesterol
Exchanges: ½ fruit

MAYONNAISE

¼ cup egg substitute
1 egg white
1⅛ teaspoons dry mustard
Dash cayenne pepper
2 tablespoons fresh lemon juice
1 tablespoon white vinegar or rice vinegar
¾ teaspoon fructose
⅔ cup plus 1 tablespoon corn oil

Combine egg substitute, egg white, mustard, cayenne pepper, lemon juice, vinegar, fructose and ⅓ cup of the oil in a blender container and blend at high speed until smooth. With blender motor running, gradually add remaining oil in a fine, steady stream, blending until mixture emulsifies and thickens. Chill 1 hour before using. Store in tightly covered jar in the refrigerator for up to 1 week. Makes 1⅓ cups.

Each 1 tablespoon serving contains about:
68 calories
8 mg sodium
8 g fat
0 mg cholesterol
Exchanges: 1¾ fat

CURRY MAYONNAISE

¾ cup low-sodium, low-calorie Mayonnaise (p. 200)
1 teaspoon curry powder
1 teaspoon fresh lemon juice
2 tablespoons grated onion
Pepper to taste

Mix together mayonnaise, curry powder, lemon juice, onion, and pepper, and blend well. Chill. Makes about ¾ cup.

Each 1 tablespoon serving contains about:
68 calories
8 mg sodium
8 g fat
0 mg cholesterol
Exchanges: 1¾ fat

MOCK HOLLANDAISE

You'll love this mock version of hollandaise when you're rushed for time—or even when you're not.

½ cup low-sodium, low-calorie Mayonnaise (p. 200)
3 tablespoons Dijon Mustard (p. 203)
2 teaspoons fresh lemon juice

Combine mayonnaise, mustard, and lemon juice in a small bowl. Blend with a wire whisk until smooth and creamy. Makes about 1 cup.

Each 1 tablespoon serving contains about:
50 calories
4 mg sodium
5 g fat
trace cholesterol
Exchanges: 1 fat

STRAWBERRY SAUCE

1½ baskets strawberries, hulled
1 tablespoon fructose
1 tablespoon fresh lemon juice

Combine strawberries, fructose, and lemon juice in a blender container and purée until smooth. Chill. Use as a topping for pies, cakes, ice cream, or puddings. Makes 1½ cups.

Each 2 tablespoon serving contains about:
14 calories
trace sodium
0 g fat
0 mg cholesterol
Exchanges: ¼ fruit

Condiments and Specialty Products

BOUQUET GARNI

Seasonal garden herbs can heighten the flavor of a saltless stock, soup, or sauce.

1 fresh sprig *each* parsley, thyme, basil, and marjoram
1 bay leaf
Celery leaves from 1 stalk
1 leaf tarragon
2 cloves garlic, split

Place parsley, thyme, basil, marjoram, bay leaf, celery tops, tarragon, and garlic in a cheesecloth square. Fold to form a bag and tie with string. Use as seasoning for sauces and soups.
NOTE: If using dried herbs, combine a pinch each of the suggested herbs in dried form. Place in cheesecloth square, fold, and tie.

Calories and sodium negligible; 0 mg cholesterol and fat

CATSUP

¾ cup low-sodium tomato juice
3 cups low-sodium tomato paste
¼ cup wine vinegar
2 cloves garlic, minced
1 teaspoon fructose

Combine tomato juice, paste, vinegar, garlic, and fructose in a mixing bowl and blend well. Refrigerate to blend flavors. Store in jars with tight-fitting lids up to 1 month in the refrigerator. Makes 1 quart.

Each 1 tablespoon serving contains about:
10 calories
5 mg sodium
0 g fat
0 mg cholesterol
Exchanges: negligible

DIJON MUSTARD

An excellent seasoning for broccoli, Brussels sprouts, cabbage, cauliflower, or greens. Try it as a marinade for beef or lamb, too.

1 cup white vinegar or rice vinegar
1 cup dry white wine
2 cups dry vermouth
1 cup finely chopped onion
2 cloves garlic, minced
1 (4-ounce) can dry mustard
2 tablespoons honey
2 teaspoons fructose
1 tablespoon vegetable oil
¼ teaspoon aromatic bitters

Combine vinegar, wine, vermouth, onion, and garlic in a saucepan and heat to boiling. Reduce heat and simmer 5 minutes. Remove from heat and cool. Strain wine mixture through a fine sieve. Put dry

Sauces, Condiments, and Specialty Recipes   203

mustard in a saucepan and pour one-fourth of the wine mixture into it, beating constantly with a wire whisk or electric mixer until smooth. Beat in remaining wine mixture, then blend in honey, fructose, oil, and bitters. Heat slowly, stirring constantly, until mixture thickens, about 10 minutes. Do not boil. Remove from heat and let cool. Pour into a glass or plastic (nonmetal) container. Cover and refrigerate at least 2 days to allow flavors to blend. Store in the refrigerator up to 3 months. Makes about 1 quart.

   Each 1 tablespoon serving contains about:
   18 calories
   trace sodium
   trace fat
   trace cholesterol
   Exchanges: negligible

CHOLESTEROL-FREE EGG SUBSTITUTE

   1 pinch saffron threads
   ¼ cup nonfat milk
   1 tablespoon nonfat milk powder
   1 teaspoon vegetable oil
   3 egg whites

Crush saffron threads to a powder with the back of a spoon. Add milk and stir to dissolve saffron. Add nonfat milk powder and vegetable oil. Beat egg whites lightly with a fork. Add milk mixture to egg whites and beat until well blended. Cover and store in the refrigerator up to 3 days. Stir well before using. Makes 6 tablespoons.
   NOTE: A dash of egg yolk can be substituted for the saffron.

   A 3-tablespoon serving contains about:
   61 calories
   102 mg sodium
   2 g fat
   1 mg cholesterol
   Exchanges: 1 meat

FRESH CRANBERRY RELISH

1 large orange
¼ cup fructose
1 tablespoon grated orange peel
1 pound fresh cranberries (4 cups)

Peel orange and cut into pieces, removing seeds and connecting membranes. Put orange pieces in a blender container with fructose and grated orange peel and blend well. Add cranberries, a few at a time, until all berries have been blended into a fairly coarse relish. Refrigerate in a covered jar several days to ripen. Serve the relish with meat or fowl, or spread on bread. Makes 4 cups.

Each ½ cup serving contains about:
29 calories
trace sodium
0 g fat
0 mg cholesterol
Exchanges: ½ fruit

HEAVENLY WHIPPED TOPPING

This low-calorie, low-fat topping made with gelatin has slightly more than half the calories of whipped cream. The flavor will fool you, too.

½ teaspoon unflavored gelatin
¼ cup cold water
4 teaspoons fructose
Whites of 2 large eggs
¼ teaspoon cream of tartar, or
½ teaspoon white vinegar
1 teaspoon vanilla extract
2 tablespoons whipped cream

Soften gelatin in cold water. Combine with fructose in a small saucepan and heat for 1½ minutes, stirring constantly, until gelatin is dissolved and the mixture is hot but not simmering. With an electric mixer on high speed, beat egg whites and cream of tartar in the top pan of a double boiler off the heat until frothy.

Heat gelatin mixture again until it starts to simmer; do not boil. Slowly pour hot gelatin mixture in a thin stream into the egg whites, beating at high speed until stiff peaks form. Beat over hot water in double boiler 1 minute. Transfer whipped topping to a bowl and place in bowl of ice water. Add vanilla extract and beat 3 minutes longer, or until the meringue just begins to set. Fold in whipped cream, a tablespoon at a time. Keep the mixture cool over ice; do not refrigerate or topping will start to weep. The topping keeps without melting for 1 hour. Just before serving, beat again gently with a rubber spatula. Makes 2½ cups.

Each 1 tablespoon serving contains about:
8 calories
10 mg sodium
trace fat
2 mg cholesterol
Exchanges: negligible

HERB BLEND

1 teaspoon *each* dried basil, marjoram, thyme,
   oregano, parsley, summer savory, ground
   cloves, mace, and black pepper
¼ teaspoon *each* ground nutmeg and
   cayenne pepper

Combine basil, marjoram, thyme, oregano, parsley, summer savory, cloves, mace, black pepper, nutmeg, and cayenne pepper in a jar with a tight-fitting lid. Store in a cool place up to 6 months. Use as seasoning for meats and vegetables. Makes about ¼ cup.

Each ¼ cup contains about:
0 calories
trace sodium
0 g fat
0 mg cholesterol
Exchanges: negligible

LOW-CALORIE MARGARINE

Low-calorie margarine is essentially margarine whipped with water. To save money, make your own. It is necessary to use at least three cups of margarine to incorporate the water completely.

> **3 cups regular or unsalted margarine, chilled**
> **3 tablespoons nonfat milk powder**
> **1½ cups ice water**

Place the margarine, milk powder, and water in a food processor or blender container and whip until water is well incorporated and margarine is light and fluffy. (You will need to turn the blender on and off, scraping mixture into blades when off.) Store in a covered plastic container for 2 to 3 weeks, or freeze for up to 3 months. Use as you would regular margarine. Makes about 6 cups.

NOTE: For each additional cup of margarine you wish to whip, add ½ cup water.

Each tablespoon of low-calorie margarine contains about:
  51 calories
  70 mg sodium (1 mg, if unsalted)
  6 g fat
  0 protein
  0 carbohydrate
  0 cholesterol

LOW-CALORIE BUTTER
Whipped Butter

Substitute unsalted butter for margarine in the above recipe.

Each tablespoon contains about:
  50 calories
  1 mg sodium
  5 g fat
  13 mg cholesterol
  Exchanges: 1 fat

CREAM CHEESE

Now you can make your own with about half the calories of regular cream cheese.

> 1 cup ricotta cheese (made from
>   partially skimmed milk)
> ½ cup low-fat cottage cheese
> ¼ cup low-fat plain yogurt
> 1 tablespoon buttermilk, or as needed

Combine ricotta cheese, cottage cheese, and yogurt in a blender container or food processor and blend well. Add buttermilk as needed for cream cheese consistency. Store refrigerated up to 1 week. Makes 1¾ cups.

> Each tablespoon contains about:
> 20 calories
> 33 mg sodium
> trace fat
> 3 mg cholesterol
> Exchanges: ¼ milk

SEAFOOD COCKTAIL SAUCE

> ¾ cup Catsup (p. 203), or
>   1 (12½-ounce) bottle low-sodium catsup
> ¼ cup fresh lemon juice, or juice of 1 large lemon
> ¼ cup minced onion
> ½ cup minced celery
> ¼ cup minced cilantro (fresh coriander) or parsley
> 4 drops hot pepper sauce
> 2 drops Worcestershire sauce
> 2 teaspoons dry horseradish
> 1 (16-ounce) can low-sodium tomato purée*

Combine Catsup, lemon juice, onion, celery, cilantro, hot pepper sauce, Worcestershire sauce, horseradish and tomato purée. Chill. Store refrigerated up to 1 week. Makes 3 cups.

*To make your own low-sodium tomato purée, place fresh peeled tomatoes or canned low-sodium tomatoes in a blender container and blend until smooth.

Each ¼ cup serving contains about:
20 calories
13 mg sodium
0 g fat
0 mg cholesterol
Exchanges: negligible

SOY SAUCE

Soy sauce diluted with broth reduces sodium content, but not flavor.

3 tablespoons mild soy sauce*
1½ cups low-sodium Beef Stock (p. 39)
¼ cup water, or
3 tablespoons strained fresh lemon juice
1 teaspoon grated lemon peel (optional)

Combine soy sauce, beef broth, water, and lemon peel. To store, refrigerate in a jar with a tight-fitting lid up to 2 weeks. Makes about 2 cups.

*Kikkoman milder soy sauce has a lower sodium content than other brands that we know of.

Each tablespoon contains about:
3 calories
60 mg sodium
trace fat
trace cholesterol
Exchanges: negligible

TARTAR SAUCE

1 cup low-sodium, low-calorie mayonnaise
1 tablespoon fresh lemon juice
2 tablespoons chopped fresh dill, or
    1 teaspoon dill weed
1½ teaspoons minced parsley
1 tablespoon minced onion
2 dashes hot pepper sauce

In a small bowl, combine mayonnaise, lemon juice, dill, parsley, onion, and hot pepper sauce. Blend together until smooth. Chill at least 1 hour before serving. Makes 1½ cups.

Each 1 tablespoon serving contains about:
    45 calories
    43 mg sodium
    5 g fat
    4 mg cholesterol
    Exchanges: 1 fat

Desserts

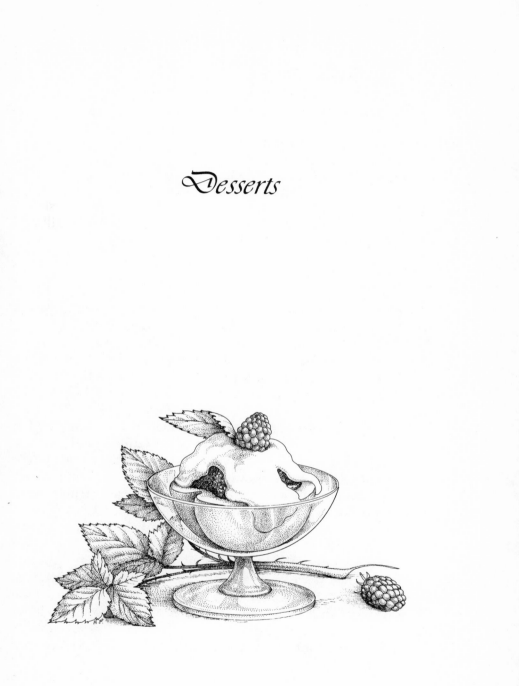

$\mathcal{W}$ell, here comes *"le pièce de résistance"*: the Dessert chapter filled with *Light Style*, light-hearted desserts that show you can have your cake and eat it, too!"

It's all there. The glamor, the flavor, the low, low (as low as we could get them) calories. A Chocolate Mousse Pie with only 184 calories per serving? A comparable piece of pie you buy in the store has triple the calories. A soufflé with negligible cholesterol? Of course. That's because we've developed one without egg yolks.

We've tried, in other words, to think of every conceivable need in designing these recipes. We use fructose to reduce total calories, seldom add any fat, and never any salt. Yet their sinfully rich flavor and taste will never convince your friends of their dietary limitations.

We've given many dessert recipes using fruit, because fruit is naturally low in calories and extra high in vitamins C and A and even fiber. It also is naturally sugared by nature, which helps keep extra calories out. Besides, they're pretty, too.

Our *Light Style* desserts show you how you can lower calories, fats, and sugar. Low-calorie margarine is substituted for butter; egg whites or egg substitute replaces egg yolks. Fructose has only half the calories of sugar and nonfat dairy products replace those high in fat content to reduce calories by half.

It won't be difficult to apply these principles to your own recipes once you've worked with ours.

212

Pies, Cakes, and Cookies

BAKLAVA

No one believes that the calories of this exquisitely light, but rich-tasting, baklava could possibly be as low as they are. But they are, thanks to *Light Style* reduction of fats, sugar, and of nuts. Rosewater Syrup, which laces the baklava, is made with fructose (half the calories of sugar because you use less) and a fraction of the margarine you would normally use. The results will fool anyone.

We thank Chef Mo Ezzani of Yemen for developing this treasured recipe for us.

    ½ pound shelled pistachio nuts, ground
    1 tablespoon fructose
    ¾ teaspoon ground cinnamon
 1½ tablespoons rosewater
    ½ pound filo dough
    ½ cup low-calorie margarine, melted
    Rosewater Syrup (following recipe)
    Whole cloves

Combine pistachio nuts, fructose, cinnamon, and rosewater in a small bowl. Using half the filo sheets (cover remaining sheets with moistened towel to prevent them from drying out), place 3 sheets in bottom of a lightly greased 13-by-9-inch baking sheet. Brush with some of the margarine. Add 3 more sheets and brush with margarine. Sprinkle evenly with nuts. Lay remaining sheets over nut filling, brushing after every third sheet and the top sheet. Cut baklava at 1½-inch intervals diagonally to form a pattern of about 35 diamond shapes. Bake at 400°F 25 minutes or until golden. Place on wire rack to cool. Drizzle Rosewater Syrup evenly over top and allow to soak several hours. Stud each diamond-shaped piece with a whole clove. Makes 35 servings.

NOTE: Filo dough and rosewater are available at Middle Eastern grocery stores and gourmet food shops.

Rosewater Syrup

1 cup water
½ cup fructose
1½ tablespoons fresh lemon juice
1 teaspoon rosewater or rum extract

Combine water and fructose in a small saucepan. Bring to a boil and boil about 30 minutes. Stir in lemon juice and rosewater. Cool completely.

Each piece contains about:
54 calories
33 mg sodium
4 g fat
0 mg cholesterol
Exchanges: ½ bread, 1 fat

CALIFORNIA CHEESECAKE

1 (16-ounce) package ricotta cheese (made from
    partially skimmed milk) or low-fat cottage cheese
4 tablespoons egg substitute, or 2 eggs
¼ cup fructose
¼ cup low-fat vanilla yogurt
1¼ teaspoons grated lemon peel
1 teaspoon fresh lemon juice
2 teaspoons vanilla extract
3 egg whites
¼ teaspoon cream of tartar, or
    1 teaspoon white vinegar
Graham Cracker Crumb Crust (following recipe)
Lemon Topping (p. 215)

Combine cheese, egg substitute or eggs, fructose, vanilla yogurt, lemon peel and juice, and vanilla extract in a mixing bowl. Beat at low speed with an electric mixer until blended, then increase speed and blend until smooth. In a small bowl, beat egg whites with cream of tartar until stiff but not dry. Gently fold egg white mixture into cheese mixture. Turn into the Graham Cracker Crumb Crust and bake at 325°F for 35 minutes, or until set. Remove from the oven and cool on a wire rack. Spread Lemon Topping over pie. Chill at least 12 hours or overnight before serving. Makes 12 servings.

Graham Cracker Crumb Crust

1 cup fine graham cracker crumbs (about 10
    graham crackers), or fine zwieback crumbs
    (about 5 zwieback)
¼ teaspoon ground cinnamon
Dash ground nutmeg (optional)
2 tablespoons low-calorie margarine, melted

Combine crumbs, cinnamon, and nutmeg in a bowl. Work in melted margarine until evenly distributed. With your fingertips, press crumb mixture evenly over the bottom and sides of a nonstick 9-inch spring-form pan. (Grease pan with low-calorie margarine, if desired.) Bake at 425°F for 5 to 7 minutes, or until crumb mixture browns slightly around edges.

Lemon Topping

2 tablespoons fructose
1½ teaspoons cornstarch
⅓ cup water
2 tablespoons fresh lemon juice
1 tablespoon egg substitute, or
    1 drop of egg yolk

In a small saucepan, combine fructose, cornstarch, water, and lemon juice. Cook and stir over low heat until thickened. Remove from heat and let cool. Stir in egg substitute or egg yolk for color. Use as topping for cheesecake or other cakes.

Each serving (one-twelfth of cake) contains about:
126 calories
101 mg sodium
8 g fat
12 mg cholesterol
Exchanges: ½ milk, ½ bread, ½ fat

CHOCOLATE MOUSSE PIE

1½ cups semisweet chocolate pieces
4 tablespoons brewed coffee
1½ teaspoons orange-flavored liqueur
1½ cups egg substitute, or 8 egg yolks
1 teaspoon vanilla extract
3 egg whites
¼ teaspoon cream of tartar
1 tablespoon fructose
Chocolate Crumb Crust (following recipe)
¾ cup Heavenly Whipped Topping (p. 205)

Melt the chocolate in the top pan of a double boiler placed over simmering water and blend in coffee and liqueur. Add egg substitute, a little at a time, or egg yolks, one at a time, blending well after each addition. Stir in vanilla and let cool slightly. In a small bowl, beat egg whites with cream of tartar until soft peaks form. Add fructose and beat until stiff but not dry. Gently fold egg white mixture into chocolate mixture, blending well but lightly. Turn into Chocolate Crumb Crust. Freeze until firm. Remove from freezer 10 minutes before serving and garnish with Heavenly Whipped Topping, allowing 1 tablespoon per serving. Sprinkle with chocolate shavings or sprinkles, if desired. Makes 12 servings.

NOTE: Chocolate leaves may be added as a decorative touch.

Chocolate Crumb Crust

20 Nabisco Famous Chocolate Wafers, finely crushed
1 tablespoon plus 2 teaspoons low-calorie margarine

Work together crumbs and margarine until crumbs are moistened. With your fingertips, press crumb mixture evenly over the bottom and sides of a greased 9-inch spring-form pan. Bake at 325°F for 10 minutes. Let cool before filling.

Each serving (one-twelfth of pie) without topping contains about:
184 calories
104 mg sodium
6 g fat
0 mg cholesterol
Exchanges: 2 bread, 1 fat

OLD-FASHIONED PUMPKIN PIE

3 tablespoons egg substitute, or
   1 egg, slightly beaten
2 tablespoons plus 1 teaspoon fructose
¾ teaspoon ground cinnamon
1½ teaspoons pumpkin pie spice
1 (16-ounce) can cooked unsalted pumpkin
⅓ cup unsweetened orange juice
¾ cup evaporated nonfat milk
2 egg whites
¼ teaspoon cream of tartar
Graham Cracker Crumb Crust (p. 215)
Heavenly Whipped Topping (p. 205), optional

Combine egg substitute or egg, 2 tablespoons of the fructose, cinnamon, pumpkin pie spice, pumpkin, and orange juice in a large bowl. Beat until well blended. Gradually add milk and beat until smooth. Beat egg whites with cream of tartar until soft peaks form. Add remaining 1 teaspoon fructose and beat until stiff but not dry. Turn into crust and bake at 350°F for 60 to 65 minutes or until knife inserted in center comes out clean. Cool on wire rack. For best results, prepare the day before to allow flavors to blend. Store in refrigerator. Serve topped with Heavenly Whipped Topping, if desired. Makes 8 servings.

Each serving (one-eighth of pie) without topping contains about:
103 calories
95 mg sodium
2 g fat
trace cholesterol
Exchanges: 1 B vegetable, 1 bread

FRENCH APPLE TART

½ cup unsweetened apple juice
¼ teaspoon maple extract
¼ teaspoon ground cinnamon
2 teaspoons fructose
½ teaspoon cornstarch
3 medium tart green apples,
    peeled, cored, and thinly sliced
Pie Crust (following recipe)

In a saucepan, combine apple juice, maple extract, cinnamon, fructose, and cornstarch. Stir until blended. Cook and stir over low heat until thickened and smooth. Remove from heat, add sliced apples, and stir to coat apple slices well. Turn into pie crust, arranging apple slices pinwheel fashion. Bake at 425°F for 20 to 30 minutes, or until apples are tender and crust is browned. Makes 8 servings.

Pie Crust

¾ cup unbleached flour
¼ teaspoon *each* grated lemon peel and orange peel
3 tablespoons vegetable oil
1½ tablespoons nonfat milk

Combine flour and lemon and orange peels in a small mixing bowl. Combine oil and milk in a measuring cup, but do not stir. Add all at once to flour mixture. Mix quickly with a fork until flour mixture begins to form a ball. Roll out between sheets of waxed paper to a very thin 12-inch circle. Fit over an 8- or 9-inch pie plate or French tart pan, trimming edges. (To make individual tarts, divide the dough into 8 portions. Roll out each ball into a 5-inch circle and fit over individual 3-inch tart pans or muffin cups.) Dough may be chilled at this point. Pierce dough with a fork in several places to allow steam to escape during baking. Bake at 450°F for 5 minutes or until golden. Cool before filling.

Each serving (one-eighth of pie) contains about:
121 calories
3 mg sodium
5 g fat
0 mg cholesterol
Exchanges: ½ fruit, 1 bread, 1 fat

·CARROT CAKE

1½ cups unbleached flour, sifted
1 teaspoon baking soda
1½ teaspoons low-sodium baking powder, or
    ½ teaspoon baking powder
½ teaspoon ground nutmeg
1½ teaspoons ground cinnamon
5 tablespoons low-calorie margarine
2 tablespoons fructose
1½ tablespoons brown sugar substitute
6 tablespoons egg substitute, or 2 eggs, beaten
½ cup nonfat milk
1½ teaspoons vanilla extract
2 cups finely grated carrots (about 3 large carrots)
½ cup fresh or water-packed canned crushed
    pineapple, well drained
2 egg whites
¼ teaspoon cream of tartar
½ cup dried currants or raisins
½ cup chopped pecans

Sift together flour, baking soda, baking powder, nutmeg, and cinnamon; set aside. Cream margarine with fructose and brown sugar substitute until well blended. Add egg, milk, and vanilla extract and blend well. (Mixture will appear curdled.) Add sifted ingredients, a third at a time, blending after each addition. Fold in carrots and pineapple. Beat egg whites with cream of tartar until stiff but not dry. Fold whites gently into batter. Fold in currants and nuts. Turn mixture into a well-greased and floured 8-inch tube pan. Bake at 350°F for 50 minutes, or until wood pick comes out clean. Cool and store in the refrigerator. Best served the same day. Makes 12 servings.

Each serving contains about:
131 calories
155 mg sodium
6 g fat
trace cholesterol
Exchanges: 1 bread, 1 fruit, 1 fat

MEXICAN BREAD PUDDING

3 to 5 cups toasted French Bread cubes, or
    3½ cups stale French Bread cubes (p. 49)
¼ cup raisins, plumped in hot water
2 cups nonfat milk
2 tablespoons low-calorie margarine
1 cup unsweetened apple juice
6 tablespoons egg substitute, or 2 egg yolks
2 tablespoons fructose
1 teaspoon vanilla extract
1 teaspoon ground cinnamon
½ teaspoon ground nutmeg
Grated peel and juice of ½ lemon

Combine bread cubes and raisins in a 13-by-9-inch nonstick baking dish. In a saucepan, scald milk and add margarine. Stir until margarine melts. Add apple juice, egg substitute or egg yolks, fructose, vanilla extract, cinnamon, nutmeg, and lemon peel and juice and mix well. Pour over bread cubes in pan and mix well. Bake at 350°F for 30 minutes, or until knife inserted in center of pudding comes out clean. Makes 8 servings.

Each ½ cup serving contains about:
88 calories
78 mg sodium
3 g fat
1 mg cholesterol
Exchanges: 1 bread, ¼ milk

SNOWDROP COOKIES

3 egg whites, at room temperature
¼ teaspoon cream of tartar, or
    1 teaspoon white vinegar
1 teaspoon vanilla extract
¾ cup fructose, or ¾ cup sugar*
¼ cup semisweet chocolate chips (tiny size)

Beat egg whites until soft peaks form. Add cream of tartar and vanilla extract and beat until stiff peaks form. Add fructose, 2 tablespoons at a time, beating after each addition. Fold in chocolate chips. Drop by heaping teaspoonfuls onto an ungreased foil-lined cookie sheet and bake at 250°F for 20 to 25 minutes, or until pale cream in color. Outside of cookie will be hard; inside will be slightly soft. Makes 36 cookies.

* Sugar substitute cannot be substituted for sugar or fructose in this recipe.

Each cookie contains about:
28 calories
4 mg sodium
trace fat
trace cholesterol
Exchanges: ½ bread

PEANUT BUTTER COOKIES

⅓ cup low-calorie margarine
¼ cup plus 2 tablespoons fructose
3 tablespoons egg substitute, or 1 egg
1 cup low-sodium, cream-style peanut butter
½ teaspoon baking soda
¼ teaspoon ground cinnamon
1 teaspoon vanilla extract
1 cup sifted unbleached flour

Cream together margarine and fructose until well blended. Beat in egg substitute or egg, peanut butter, baking soda, cinnamon, and vanilla extract until smooth. Add flour and beat until well blended. Roll dough into balls about ¾-inch in diameter and place on ungreased cookie sheets. Score in crisscross fashion with fork tines to flatten. Bake at 375°F for 10 to 12 minutes or until browned. Remove cookies from sheets and cool on wire racks. Makes 80 cookies.

Each cookie contains about:
29 calories

15 mg sodium
2 g fat
0 mg cholesterol
Exchanges: ½ bread

Fruit

BERRY BOWL

3 cups strawberries, hulled and
   halved lengthwise
1 cup fresh or frozen unsweetened raspberries,
   thawed, or any berries
1 teaspoon fructose
1 tablespoon Framboise or Kirsch

Combine strawberries and raspberries in a bowl. Sprinkle with fructose and drizzle with Framboise. Toss and serve. Makes 8 servings.

Each ½ cup serving contains about:
   56 calories
   61 mg sodium
   0 g fat
   0 mg cholesterol
   Exchanges: 1 fruit

CITRUS COMPOTE

3 oranges
1 grapefruit
½ cup water
½ teaspoon vanilla extract
⅛ teaspoon ground cloves
1 tablespoon fructose
2 tablespoons raisins
Fresh mint sprigs

Grate peels of oranges and grapefruit into a saucepan. Be careful to use only color part of peels. Peel, seed, and dice oranges and grapefruit over the saucepan so no juice is lost. Add diced fruit, water, vanilla extract, cloves, fructose, and raisins to pan, bring to a boil, and simmer, uncovered, 10 minutes. Cool and chill. Spoon into stemmed glasses and garnish with mint sprigs, if desired. Makes 6 servings.

Each ½ cup serving contains about:
  60 calories
  61 mg sodium
  0 g fat
  0 mg cholesterol
  Exchanges: 1 fruit

PAPAYA WITH LIME

3 papayas
Juice of 2 limes
6 lime wedges
Fresh mint sprigs

Peel and halve papayas. Remove seeds and discard. Place each papaya half, cut side down, on a serving plate. Slice horizontally ¼ inch thick and fan out slices slightly on plate. Sprinkle slices with lime juice and garnish with lime wedges and mint sprigs. Makes 6 servings.

Each serving contains about:
  44 calories
  4 mg sodium
  0 g fat
  0 mg cholesterol
  Exchanges: 1 fruit

PEACHES GALLIANO

3 cups peeled and sliced peaches
  (6 small peaches)
½ cup fresh or frozen unsweetened
  blueberries, thawed
1 tablespoon Galliano

Place peach slices in a bowl. Top with blueberries and sprinkle with Galliano. Toss just before serving. Makes 6 servings.

Each ½ cup serving contains about:
  54 calories
  1 mg sodium
  0 g fat
  0 mg cholesterol
  Exchanges: 1 fruit

PEACH MELBA

3 peaches, peeled, pitted, and halved, or
  6 canned water-packed peach halves
6 tablespoons puréed raspberries
6 tablespoons low-fat vanilla yogurt

Place a peach half in each of six parfait glasses. Put 1 tablespoon raspberry purée on each peach. Top each with a tablespoon of yogurt. Makes 6 servings.

Each serving contains about:
  45 calories
  13 mg sodium
  1 g fat
  1 mg cholesterol
  Exchanges: 1 fruit

PEARS ALEXANDER

This quick-change artist triples as an appetizer, salad, or dessert.

>   6 small ripe pears, or
>   12 canned water-packed pear halves
>   1 tablespoon fresh lemon juice
>   ½ cup ricotta cheese (made from partially
>   skimmed milk), at room temperature
>   2 tablespoons Cream Cheese (p. 208)
>   1 tablespoon golden raisins
>   3 tablespoons crushed pistachio nuts,
>   pecans, or walnuts

If using fresh pears, peel and cut each pear in half lengthwise, leaving stems intact on one pear half. Core centers to form cavities. Brush pears with lemon juice to prevent discoloration. Beat ricotta and cream cheeses with a wooden spoon until soft and fluffy. Mix in raisins. Fill each pear cavity with about 1 tablespoon cheese mixture and then put pear halves together to form whole pears. Sprinkle in crushed nuts. Arrange on a serving plate and chill 2 hours before serving. If desired, cut pears horizontally into ½-inch slices to serve over a bed of lettuce for salad or first-course appetizer. Makes 6 servings.

>   Each serving contains about:
>   128 calories
>   31 mg sodium (content unavailable for pistachio nuts)
>   7 g fat
>   5 mg cholesterol
>   Exchanges: 1 fruit, 1 fat

PINEAPPLE IN RUM

Freeze the spears and you'll have edible swizzle sticks for tall summery drinks.

> 1 small pineapple, peeled, cored, and
>   cut lengthwise in 12 spears
> 2 tablespoons rum
> Fresh mint sprigs

Marinate pineapple spears in rum, tossing frequently, at least 2 hours or overnight. Allow 2 spears per serving. Place on dessert plates and garnish with mint sprigs. Makes 6 servings.

Each serving contains about:
40 calories
1 mg sodium
0 g fat
0 mg cholesterol
Exchanges: 1 fruit

STRAWBERRIES IN MERINGUE

> 1 basket strawberries, hulled and
>   halved lengthwise
> Meringue Shells (following recipe)
> Heavenly Whipped Topping (p. 205)

Arrange sliced strawberries, point up, in Meringue Shells. Top each with 1 tablespoon Heavenly Whipped Topping. Makes 6 servings.

Meringue Shells

> 3 egg whites, at room temperature
> 1 teaspoon cream of tartar
> 1 teaspoon vanilla extract
> ¾ cup fructose, or ¾ cup sugar

Beat egg whites until soft peaks form. Add cream of tartar and vanilla and beat until stiff. Add fructose, 2 tablespoons at a time beating after each addition. For each shell, drop 2 heaping tablespoons of egg white mixture on a foil-lined baking sheet. Make indentations to form shells. Bake at 250°F for 30 to 35 minutes, or until pale golden in color. Outside will be hard and inside soft. Cool, then remove from baking sheet. Makes 6 shells.

Each serving contains about:
  97 calories
  5 mg sodium
  trace fat
  0 mg cholesterol
  Exchanges: 1 fruit

STRAWBERRIES ROMANOFF

1 teaspoon rum extract or, 1 tablespoon rum
1 cup Heavenly Whipped Topping (p. 205)
¼ cup vanilla yogurt
2 baskets ripe strawberries, hulled and
    sliced or left whole

Stir rum into Heavenly Whipped Topping, then blend in vanilla yogurt. Chill until serving time. Spoon ½ cup berries in each of 6 stemmed sherbet glasses. Top with about 3 tablespoons of the topping. Makes 6 servings.

Each ½ cup strawberries with 3 tablespoons topping
contains about:
  57 calories
  32 mg sodium
  trace fat
  trace cholesterol
  Exchanges: 1 fruit

MELON BASKETS

3 small cantaloupes
2 cups watermelon balls
2 cups honeydew melon balls
2 tablespoons orange-flavored liqueur
Fresh mint sprigs

Cut cantaloupes in half. Scoop out seeds and carve balls from flesh, leaving cantaloupe shells intact. Combine cantaloupe balls with watermelon and honeydew in a bowl. Drizzle with liqueur and toss to blend flavors. Place 1 cup melon balls in each of the 6 cantaloupe shells. Garnish with mint sprigs. Makes 6 servings.

Each serving contains about:
62 calories
8 mg sodium
0 g fat
0 mg cholesterol
Exchanges: 1 fruit

BERRIES ON ICE

24 long-stemmed strawberries
Crushed ice
2 tablespoons brown sugar
2 tablespoons low-fat plain yogurt

Attractively arrange strawberries on a bed of crushed ice in a bowl. Place brown sugar in one small bowl and the yogurt in another. Dip strawberries first in sugar and then in yogurt to eat. Makes 6 servings.

Each serving (4 strawberries with dips) contains about:
33 calories
3 mg sodium
trace fat
trace cholesterol
Exchanges: ½ fruit

Ices and Ice Creams

COFFEE ICE

1 envelope (1 tablespoon) unflavored gelatin
¼ cup water
2 cups hot strong coffee
¼ cup plus 2 teaspoons fructose
Juice of 2 lemons and 1 orange
1 teaspoon *each* grated lemon and
    orange peels

Soften gelatin in water, then dissolve in hot coffee. Add fructose, juices, and peels. Turn into a bowl or freezer tray and freeze until slushy. Beat until evenly blended, return to freezer, and freeze until almost solid. Break up ice and beat until slushy. Return to freezer and freeze solid. Remove from freezer 20 minutes before serving time. Chop with a spoon until mixture is consistency of thick slush. Spoon into serving dishes. Makes 1 quart.

    Each ½ cup serving contains about:
      33 calories
      trace sodium
      0 g fat
      0 mg cholesterol
      Exchanges: ½ bread

STRAWBERRY ICE

1 envelope (1 tablespoon) unflavored gelatin
1 cup water
2 teaspoons fructose
2 cups Strawberry Sauce (p. 202)
1 teaspoon fresh lemon juice

Soften gelatin in ¼ cup of the water. Heat remaining ¾ cup water and add fructose and gelatin mixture, stirring until gelatin dissolves.

Remove from heat and cool. Stir in Strawberry Sauce and lemon juice. Turn into a bowl or freezer tray and freeze until slushy. Beat until evenly blended, return to freezer, and freeze until almost solid. Break up ice and beat until slushy. Return to freezer and freeze solid. Remove from freezer 20 minutes before serving. Chop with a spoon until mixture is consistency of thick slush. Spoon into serving dishes. Makes about 3 cups.

Each ½ cup serving contains about:
44 calories
trace sodium
0 g fat
0 mg cholesterol
Exchanges: 1 fruit

VANILLA ICE CREAM

This ice cream has half the calories and fat of the commercial ones.

3½ cups evaporated nonfat milk
¼ cup plus 1 tablespoon fructose
1½ teaspoons vanilla extract

Combine the evaporated milk, fructose, and vanilla. Put in an ice cream freezer and freeze according to manufacturer's directions. Makes about 5 cups.

Each ½ cup serving contains about:
84 calories
115 mg sodium
1 g fat
trace cholesterol
Exchanges: ½ milk, 1 fruit

Apricot or Peach Ice Cream

Use 4 pounds ripe apricots or peaches. Peel, pit, slice, and purée the fruit. Fold it into Vanilla Ice Cream mixture (preceding recipe) at midpoint of freezing, then finish freezing. Makes about 1½ quarts.

Strawberry Ice Cream

Prepare Strawberry Sauce (p. 202) and fold into Vanilla Ice Cream mixture (p. 230) at midpoint of freezing, then finish freezing.

Each ½ cup serving strawberry, apricot, or peach ice cream contains about:
  90 calories
  115 mg sodium
  1 g fat
  trace cholesterol
  Exchanges: ½ milk, 1 fruit

Sweet Crêpes

APPLE SIZZLE CREPES

1 tablespoon low-calorie margarine
2 medium tart green apples or
    Golden Delicious apples, peeled, cored, and
    thinly sliced
½ cup unsweetened apple juice
2 teaspoons cornstarch
1 teaspoon fructose
¼ teaspoon *each* vanilla extract and
    maple extract
1 teaspoon water
6 Feather Crêpes (p. 69)
Heavenly Whipped Topping (p. 205)
Ground cinnamon
Toasted almonds (optional)

In a skillet, melt margarine over low heat. Add apples and apple juice and mix gently. Cover and cook over low heat until apples are soft, stirring occasionally, about 10 minutes. Mix cornstarch with fructose, vanilla and maple extracts, and water. Stir into apple mixture and cook and stir until apple mixture thickens. Top each crêpe with ¼ cup apple filling. Roll jelly-roll fashion and serve topped with 2 tablespoons Heavenly Whipped Topping. Sprinkle with cinnamon and toasted almonds, if desired. Makes 6 servings.

Strawberry Crêpes

Fill each Feather Crêpe with ¼ cup sliced strawberries. Roll jelly-roll fashion and top with 1 tablespoon low-fat plain yogurt and 2 tablespoons Strawberry Sauce (p. 202).

Peach Crêpes

Fill each Feather Crêpe with ¼ cup sliced peaches. Roll jelly-roll fashion and top with 2 tablespoons low-fat peach yogurt.

Each apple, strawberry, or peach crêpe contains about:
  57 calories (apples), 72 (strawberries), 86 (peaches)
  20 mg sodium
  trace g fat
  trace cholesterol
  Exchanges: ½ fruit, ½ bread

FRUIT IN CREPE BASKETS

  1 medium banana, diagonally sliced
  ½ teaspoon fresh lemon juice
  1 cup fresh or unsweetened frozen blueberries or
      blackberries, thawed
  1 cup sliced strawberries
  ½ cup melon balls or cubes
  6 Feather Crêpe Cups (p. 70)
  6 tablespoons low-fat fruit-flavored
      yogurt of choice
  1 kiwi fruit, peeled and sliced (optional)

Place banana slices in a large bowl. Sprinkle with lemon juice to prevent darkening. Add berries and melon balls and toss to blend flavors. Place ½ cup of the fruit mixture in each crêpe cup. Top with 1 tablespoon yogurt and garnish with a slice of kiwi fruit, if available, or other cut fruit. Makes 6 servings.

Each crêpe cup with ½ cup fruit contains about:
73 calories
43 mg sodium
1 g fat
trace cholesterol
Exchanges: ½ bread, 1 fruit

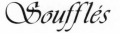

CHOCOLATE SOUFFLE

1 tablespoon cornstarch
1 tablespoon fructose
½ cup nonfat milk
¼ cup evaporated nonfat milk
3 squares (3 ounces) semisweet chocolate, broken
1 tablespoon crème de cacao
½ cup egg substitute, or 3 eggs
3 egg whites
¼ teaspoon cream of tartar or 1 teaspoon vinegar

Combine cornstarch, fructose, and milks in a saucepan. Bring to a boil, reduce heat to low, and cook and stir until thickened and smooth. Add chocolate and crème de cacao. Remove from heat and stir until chocolate melts. Cool slightly. Mix in egg substitute, a tablespoon at a time, or eggs, one at a time. Beat egg whites with cream of tartar until stiff but not dry. Stir one-fourth of whites into chocolate sauce to lighten it, then gently fold in remaining whites. Spoon into six individual greased ½-cup soufflé dishes or a greased 1-quart soufflé dish and bake at 350°F for 10 to 15 minutes for individual soufflés and 40 minutes for large, or until set and puffy. Do not overcook. Serve at once. Makes 6 servings.

Each ½ cup serving contains about:
   124 calories
   48 mg sodium
   8 g fat
   1 mg cholesterol
   Exchanges: 1 bread, 1¼ fat

LEMON SOUFFLE

The staying power of this lemony soufflé is amazing.

   ½ cup evaporated nonfat milk
   ¼ cup water
   4½ teaspoons cornstarch
   5 tablespoons fresh lemon juice
   2 teaspoons grated lemon peel
   ½ cup egg substitute, or 4 egg yolks
   2 egg whites
   ¼ teaspoon cream of tartar, or
          1 teaspoon vinegar
   ¼ cup fructose

Combine milk, water, and cornstarch in small saucepan. Bring to a
boil, reduce heat to low, and cook and stir until sauce is thickened
and smooth. Remove from heat and stir in lemon juice and peel.
Cool slightly. Mix in egg substitute, a tablespoon at a time, or egg
yolks, one at a time. Beat egg whites with cream of tartar until stiff
but not dry. Beat in fructose. Stir one-fourth of whites into lemon
sauce to lighten it, then gently fold in remaining whites. Turn into a
greased 1-quart soufflé dish or casserole. Bake at 350°F for 45
minutes, or until set and puffy. Do not overcook. Serve at once.
Makes 6 servings.

   Each ½ cup serving contains about
      81 calories
      90 mg sodium
      4 g fat
      trace cholesterol
      Exchanges: ½ bread, ½ fruit, 1 fat

STRAWBERRY SOUFFLE

1 basket strawberries, hulled
2 teaspoons fresh lemon juice
2 tablespoons cornstarch
2 tablespoons water
3 tablespoons fructose
6 tablespoons egg substitute, or 2 egg yolks
2 egg whites
¼ teaspoon cream of tartar, or
      1 teaspoon white vinegar

Purée strawberries, reserving 4 large whole berries. Mix purée with lemon juice in a saucepan. Finely dice the 4 reserved berries and add to purée. Dissolve cornstarch in water. Add to saucepan with fructose. Bring to a boil, reduce heat to low, and cook and stir until smooth and thickened, about 2 to 3 minutes. Cool slightly. Mix in egg substitute, a tablespoon at a time, or egg yolks, one at a time. Beat egg whites with cream of tartar until stiff but not dry. Stir one-fourth of whites into strawberry sauce to lighten it, then gently fold in remaining whites. Turn into a greased 1-quart soufflé dish or casserole and bake at 375°F 30 minutes, or until set and puffy. Serve at once. Makes 6 servings.

    Each ½ cup serving contains about:
    60 calories
    73 mg sodium
    2 g fat
    0 mg cholesterol
    Exchanges: 1 fruit

Beverages

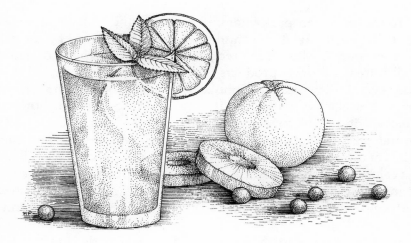

$\mathcal{B}$everages can be deceptively high in calories and often the culprit in pushing your daily calorie limits over the edge.

A couple of 12-ounce glasses of regular beer, consumed each evening, can add 300 calories a day. That's 2,100 calories or more than one-half pound body weight added each week. An eggnog sipped at a party will add 250 calories to an already calorie-loaded holiday meal.

You actually can pack vitamins A and C and unload calories in your diet each day, if you think of beverages as part of your daily nutrient intake. Most of the recipes that follow make use of natural fruit juices and dairy products for maximum nutrition. There are also several recipes using alcoholic beverages. You'll get half the calories of a glass of wine by diluting it with club soda, however. Calories of a drink made with dairy products also go down when nonfat products are used. Relying on the natural-occurring sugar effect of unsweetened fruit juices and fruits instead of sugar will help cut calories, too. Egg substitute replaces eggs for an 86-calorie cup of eggnog. You won't get the high nutritional value of a drink made with eggs, but you'll know how to cut calories when they become a problem.

So cheers! We think you'll enjoy our low-calorie, low-fat, low-sodium drinks. There are punches for parties, smoothies that wake you up, and nightcaps that bed you down. There are a few beverages that children will enjoy with their cookies, and an herb tea grandma will love to share with friends.

238

BLOODY MARY

1 quart low-sodium tomato juice
Dash hot pepper sauce
Pepper to taste
1 teaspoon fresh lemon juice
¼ teaspoon *each* onion powder and
      Worcestershire sauce
3 jiggers vodka
Ice cubes
6 celery stalks with leaves

Combine the tomato juice, hot pepper sauce, pepper, lemon juice, onion powder, Worcestershire sauce, and vodka in a pitcher. Stir to blend well. Pour in individual glasses over ice. Add celery stalk, leaf side up. Makes 6 servings.

    Each ¾ cup serving contains about:
    67 calories
    33 mg sodium
    0 g fat
    0 mg cholesterol
    Exchanges: 1 B vegetable

Virgin Mary

Follow directions for Bloody Mary (preceding recipe) but omit the vodka. Nutrient analysis is the same as for Bloody Mary, except calories are reduced to 32 per serving.

BREAKFAST SHAKE

All you need is some toast to complete this breakfast-in-a-glass.

1 cup nonfat milk
2 heaping teaspoons sweetened cocoa powder
3 tablespoons egg substitute, or 1 egg
1 small banana

Combine milk, cocoa, egg substitute and banana in a blender container. Blend until frothy and smooth. Makes 1 serving.

Each serving contains about:
270 calories
199 mg sodium
6 g fat
5 mg cholesterol
Exchanges: 1 milk, 1 meat, 1 fruit, ¼ bread

EGGNOG

4 cups nonfat milk
1 cup egg substitute, or 6 eggs
2½ tablespoons fructose
2 or 3 teaspoons rum extract
2 egg whites
About 2 tablespoons Heavenly Whipped
    Topping (p. 205)
Ground nutmeg

Combine milk, egg substitute or eggs, 2 tablespoons of the fructose, and rum extract in a bowl. Beat with rotary beater or electric mixer until well blended. Chill thoroughly. Beat egg whites lightly with remaining fructose and fold into milk mixture. Top each serving with 1 teaspoon Heavenly Whipped Topping and sprinkle with nutmeg. Makes 8 servings.

Each 5 ounce serving contains about:
86 calories
83 mg sodium
4 g fat
2 mg cholesterol
Exchanges: 1 milk

HERB TEA

No calories, cholesterol, or sodium in this tea, so enjoy it as a refreshment any time of the day.

Water
Lemon, orange and/or mint leaves
Cinnamon stick (optional)

Using ¾ cup of water per cup of tea, bring water to a boil. For each serving, add 3 lemon, orange, or mint leaves, or a combination, to the boiling water. Cover, turn off the heat, and steep for 2 to 3 minutes. (The longer the leaves steep, the stronger the tea.) For additional flavor, add ½ cinnamon stick to leaves while brewing.

Sodium is negligible; no calories or cholesterol.

MIMOSA COCKTAIL

1 fifth Champagne
4 cups unsweetened orange juice
Ice cubes
Orange slices
Fresh mint leaves

Fill stemmed wine glasses or goblets with half Champagne and half orange juice. Add ice cubes and garnish with orange slices and mint leaves. Makes about 8 servings.

Each 8 ounce serving contains about:
110 calories
1 mg sodium
0 g fat
0 mg cholesterol
Exchanges: 1 fruit, ½ bread

PERSIAN REFRESHER

1 quart buttermilk*
1 teaspoon dried mint, or
   1 tablespoon chopped fresh mint
Ice cubes
Fresh mint sprigs (optional)

Mix buttermilk with dried or chopped mint. Pour over ice cubes in tall glasses. Garnish with mint sprigs, if desired. Makes 6 servings.

*Note that buttermilk is high in sodium and, if you must watch sodium intake, substitute plain low-fat yogurt.

Each 5 ounce serving contains about:
59 calories
212 mg sodium
1 g fat
3 mg cholesterol
Exchanges: ¾ milk

SPARKLING PUNCH

Unsweetened cranberry juice
Lime-flavored carbonated beverage (sugar-free), or
   club soda
Ice Ring (following recipe)
Orange slices
Fresh mint sprigs

Combine equal parts cranberry juice and lime beverage in a punch bowl. Add Ice Ring and float orange slices and mint sprigs on top of punch.

Ice Ring

Fill ring mold with distilled water to within ¼ inch of rim. Freeze until solid. Dip briefly in hot water to unmold and place in punch bowl.

Each 8 ounce serving contains about:
  20 calories
  18 mg sodium
  0 g fat
  0 mg cholesterol
  Exchanges: ½ fruit

SUNRISE PUNCH

1 quart unsweetened cranberry juice
1 quart unsweetened orange juice
1 quart unsweetened pineapple juice
Orange slices
Fresh mint sprigs

Combine cranberry juice, orange juice, and pineapple juice and stir well to blend. Pour into glasses and garnish each serving with an orange slice and a mint sprig. Makes about 25 servings.

Each 4 ounce serving contains about:
  60 calories
  trace sodium
  0 g fat
  0 mg cholesterol
  Exchanges: 1 fruit

WINE SPRITZER

1 quart club soda
1 quart dry white or red wine
Ice cubes
Lime or lemon wedges

Put ½ cup club soda and ½ cup wine in each of 8 tall glasses. Add ice cubes and garnish with lime wedges. Makes 8 servings.

Each 8 ounce serving contains about:
  84 calories

37 mg sodium
0 g fat
0 mg cholesterol
Exchanges: 1 bread

Virgin Spritzer

Substitute 1 quart unsweetened orange juice for the wine in Wine Spritzer. Makes 8 servings.

Each 8 ounce serving contains about:
56 calories
32 mg sodium
0 g fat
0 mg cholesterol
Exchanges: 1 fruit

YOGURT SMOOTHIE

**½ cup frozen or chilled low-fat
fruit-flavored or plain yogurt
½ cup nonfat milk
½ cup fresh or unsweetened canned fruit, drained**

Combine yogurt, milk and fruit. Blend until smooth. Makes 2 servings.

Each 6 ounce serving contains about:
200 calories
135 mg sodium
2 g fat
6 mg cholesterol
Exchanges: ½ milk, ¼ fruit

NOTE: For a nutritionally rich Smoothie, add 2 tablespoons of 1 beaten egg, and blend. Calories will increase to 280, sodium to 188 mg, cholesterol to 228 mg, and fat to 7 g.

Menus

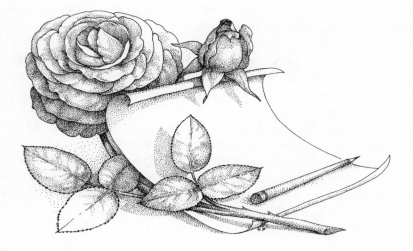

$\mathcal{S}$tudies show that most people have difficulty preparing menus. A menu balanced in nutrients, low in calories, fats, cholesterol, salt, and sugar, yet glamorous, quick, and easy to prepare is a tall order. It takes skill and experience and knowledge about nutrients to fill the order.

Our menu suggestions take all the guesswork out of menu planning. Plus, the nutrient analysis included with each menu shows you at a glance the amount of sodium, fats, cholesterol, and calories each person is getting. This will help you plan meals according to individual or family needs.

That doesn't mean you may not stray from the menu suggestions. We hope they will be used as a guide for further menu planning. If you substitute dishes, you will know the exact nutrient content of each dish because each recipe contains an analysis. These analyses for the complete menu will help you make wise food choices. And that, after all, is the goal of this chapter.

BARBECUE BASH
Pizza Canapes (p. 20)
Barbecued Chicken (p. 89)
Corn on the Cob
Marinated Mushrooms (p. 163)
Ice Cream (pp. 230-231)

Nutrient Analysis
395 calories
350 mg sodium
10 g fat
65 mg cholesterol

FRIED CHICKEN DINNER
Oven-Fried Chicken (p. 97)
Coleslaw De Luxe (p. 160)
Oven-Fried Potatoes (p. 151)
Corn Bread (p. 47)
Melon Baskets (p. 228)

Nutrient Analysis
479 Calories
280 mg sodium
16 g fat
62 mg cholesterol

FRIDAY FISH DINNER
Skinny Dip (p. 15) with assorted vegetables
Swordfish Piquant (p. 80)
Steamed Asparagus (p. 138)
Rice Pilaf (p. 130)
Pears Alexander (p. 225)

Nutrient Analysis
435 calories
174 mg sodium
22 g fat
65 mg cholesterol

SUNDAY LASAGNA DINNER
Chicken Pacifica (p. 17)
Lasagna (p. 127)
Broccoli alla Romana (p. 139)
Marinated Mushrooms (p. 163)
California Cheesecake (p. 214)

Nutrient Analysis
471 calories
404 mg sodium
24 g fat
72 mg cholesterol

SATURDAY SUPPER
Lobster Bisque (p. 33)
Ratatouille Crêpes (p. 69)
Strawberries Romanoff (p. 227)

Nutrient Analysis
204 calories
156 mg sodium
8 g fat
41 mg cholesterol

CHINESE DINNER
Chinatown Soup (p. 29)
Chicken Oriental (p. 95)
Steamed Rice (p. 132)
Chinese Stir-Fry Vegetables (p. 141)
Melon with Port (p. 18)

Nutrient Analysis
437 calories
347 mg sodium
7 g fat
77 mg cholesterol

MEXICAN DINNER
Tortilla Salad (p. 24)
Enchiladas Suiza (p. 92)
Spanish Rice (p. 131)
Zucchini Oregano (p. 149)
Pineapple in Rum (p. 226)

Nutrient Analysis:
500 calories
133 mg sodium
14 g fat
42 mg cholesterol

FANCY ITALIAN DINNER
Appetizer Artichokes (p. 16)
Kathy's Cannelloni (p. 125)
Tomato-Cauliflower Salad (p. 165)
Peaches Galliano (p. 224)

Nutrient Analysis (Based on 2 Cannelloni per serving)
352 calories
221 mg sodium
19 g fat
42 mg cholesterol

DINNER FOR TWO OR FOUR
Chilled Crookneck Soup (p. 38)
Steak Diane (p. 111)
Green Beans Amandine (p. 142)
Pommes Parisienne (p. 152)
California Salad (p. 167)
Chocolate Soufflé (p. 233)

Nutrient Analysis
595 calories
256 mg sodium
26 g fat
84 mg cholesterol

FESTIVE HOLIDAY DINNER
Eggnog (p. 240)
Roast Turkey with Royal Glaze (p. 99)
Turkey Gravy (p. 189)
Apple-Onion Stuffing (p. 99)
Peas and Pods (p. 145)
Candied Sweets (p. 150)
Sunshine Salad (p. 172)
Cloud Biscuits (p. 45)
Old-Fashioned Pumpkin Pie (p. 217)

Nutrient Analysis
746 calories
549 mg sodium
22 g fat
74 mg cholesterol

HOLLYWOOD BOWL PICNIC
Gazpacho Andaluz (p. 39)
Picnic Lobster with Seafood Cocktail Sauce (p. 208)
Mediterranean Salad (p. 164)
Ramona's Rolls (p. 52)
Carrot Cake (p. 219)

Nutrient Analysis
405 calories
501 mg sodium
12 g fat
115 mg cholesterol

SIT-DOWN DINNER
Scallops Dejonghe (p. 20)
Cornish Game Hens with Herb-Corn Bread Stuffing (p. 101)
Green Beans Amandine (p. 142)
Endive-Watercress Salad (p. 161)
with Lemon Dressing (p. 180)
Crescent Rolls (p. 46)
Peach Melba (p. 224)

Nutrient Analysis
559 calories
554 mg sodium
15 g fat
100 mg cholesterol

SPAGHETTI DINNER
Hearty Minestrone (p. 32)
Spaghetti with Italian Meat Sauce (p. 129)
Hearts of Romaine Lettuce
Creamy Garlic Dressing (p. 178)
Lemon Spinach (p. 144)
French Bread (p. 49)
Coffee Ice (p. 229)

Nutrient Analysis
339 calories
113 mg sodium
3 g fat
32 mg cholesterol

CLUB LUNCHEON
Consommé Madrilène (p. 30)
Chicken-Stuffed Papaya (p. 169)
Bread Sticks (p. 49)
Chocolate Mousse Pie (p. 216)

Nutrient Analysis
485 calories
206 mg sodium
14 g fat
63 mg cholesterol

SUNDAY FOOTBALL TV LUNCH
Albondigas Soup (p. 27)
California Tostada (p. 158)
Papaya with Lime (p. 223)

Nutrient Analysis
501 calories
346 mg sodium
16 g fat
112 mg cholesterol

ELEGANT BRUNCH
Bloody Mary (p. 239)
Spinach Soufflé (p. 61)
Waldorf Salad (p. 170)
Ramona's Whole Wheat Bread, toasted (p. 52)
Ice Cream (pp. 230-231)

Nutrient Analysis
346 calories
401 mg sodium
11 g fat
1 mg cholesterol

FIRESIDE SUPPER
French Onion Soup (p. 31)
Omelet Supreme (p. 59)
Garlic Bread (p. 48)
French Apple Tart (p. 218)

Nutrient Analysis
391 calories
313 mg sodium
20 g fat
8 mg cholesterol

Modifying Recipes

These handy tips for substituting ingredients high in fats, calories, cholesterol, and sodium for those lower in these nutrients should help anyone successfully modify any recipe—ours or yours.

This chapter is but one of the tools of recipe modification. The entire book has been designed with modification in mind. The recipes and back matter provide you with immediate answers for substituting sweeteners to lower calories, egg substitutes to lower cholesterol, flavoring agents to replace salt, thickeners to reduce fat and calories, plus a host of others.

To some degree, recipe modification calls for experimentation. Play with the seasonings. Be daring with ingredient substitutions. Experimentation, after all, can be an adventure that not only instructs, but entertains as well.

Chocolate

Use cocoa powder instead of chocolate to reduce calories and saturated fat. For each square (1-ounce) of chocolate, use 3 tablespoons cocoa plus 1 tablespoon low-calorie margarine. Place over hot water in double boiler and cook, stirring, until smooth.

Condiments

Low-sodium condiments purchased commercially or homemade will substantially reduce sodium in recipes calling for them. Commercial soy sauce contains 1200 mg per tablespoon while *Light Style's* (p. 209) contains 60 mg per tablespoon. For Dijon Mustard, see p. 203; Catsup, p. 203; stocks, pp. 39 through 41; Low-Sodium Baking Powder, p. 289; Seafood Cocktail Sauce, p. 208.

Eggs

Egg substitute (commercial or our recipe on p. 204) can be used in place of eggs in any recipe calling for eggs to lower calories and cholesterol. Check package labels for calorie and sodium counts. Use 3 tablespoons (1½ ounces) egg substitute for each egg.

Stiffly beaten egg whites can be folded into sauces to add volume to desserts and lower calories. (See California Cheesecake, p. 214.)

Fat

You'll lower calories, cholesterol, fat, and sodium by using low-calorie margarine (our version, p. 207, or commercial).

Low-calorie mayonnaise, ours (p. 200) or commercial, will help cut the fat, sodium, and calorie content in recipes calling for mayonnaise.

You'll use less fat if you use nonstick utensils.

The use of egg substitute reduces saturated fat and cholesterol intake by eliminating fat-rich egg yolks.

Milk

Use nonfat milk in place of whole milk in recipes calling for milk to reduce total calories, fat, and cholesterol content.

Use evaporated nonfat milk instead of cream or half-and-half in recipes calling for cream to reduce calories considerably—by at least half.

Salt

Use herbs and spices in place of salt in recipes. See pages 281 to 285 for ideas on seasoning meats, fish, poultry, sauces, and vegetables with herbs and spices.

Citrus peels can point up flavors of foods cooked without salt.

Use lemon juice and wine as flavorings for unsalted foods.

Those on an extreme low-sodium diet should use low-sodium baking powder (p. 289) and other low-sodium products to help cut sodium as much as possible.

Sauces and Creams

Egg whites will add "creamy" volume to soufflés, mousses, and cakes. (See the soufflés on pages 60 through 62 and pages 233 through 235.)

Use Heavenly Whipped Topping on page 205 instead of whipped cream to thicken dessert creams and sauces. Calories, fat, and cholesterol will be reduced considerably.

For dips and spreads calling for cream cheese, use our low-calorie Cream Cheese (p. 208) or low-fat cottage cheese that has been puréed in the blender. Not only are they low in calories and fat, but loaded with nutrients.

You'll reduce calories if you use arrowroot or cornstarch in place of flour in sauces, because you need less—about half as much.

Sweeteners

Fruit (dried, fresh, or unsweetened canned) have natural sweetness. Use fruit and fruit juices to sweeten sauces. (See Apple Sizzle Crêpes, p. 231.)

Substitute fructose for sugar in recipes calling for sugar. For each cup sugar, use ½ to ¾ cup fructose. Also use manufacturers' substitution suggestions. Fructose has the same calories as sugar, but because it is 1½ times sweeter, you use less. Therefore, you reduce calories by half.

For those who must reduce sugar intake, low-calorie maple syrup is an excellent substitute for molasses (see Ramona's Whole Wheat Bread, p. 52), as are low-calorie jellies and jams as glazes for vegetables such as carrots, or for poultry (see Carrots à l'Orange, p. 139, and Roast Turkey with Royal Glaze, p. 99).

Guide to Good Eating

The Recommended Dietary Allowances grew out of concern over the fitness—or lack of it—of military men during World War II.

The panel of nutrition experts now known as the Food and Nutrition Board of the National Academy of Sciences were summoned to define nutritional requirements. Those requirements became known as the RDA (Recommended Dietary Allowances). The RDA undergoes alterations or additions every five years. However, the RDA has little meaning for the layman, except in overall terms. It takes a scientist or nutritionist to interpret the value of 1.5 milligrams riboflavin in terms of food intake.

To help translate the RDA into meaningful food recommendations, the United States Department of Agriculture determined that adults need a minimum of two (2) daily servings from the milk group, two (2) from the meat group, four (4) from the vegetable-fruit group, and four (4) from the bread-cereal group: Children, however, need 3-2-4-4 from those groups and teenagers even more—4-2-4-4, because of their growing body needs. Like growing children, pregnant women have increased dietary needs. This group needs extra or larger servings from the milk, fruit-vegetable, and meat group, with special attention to sources of protein, iron, and calcium. Teenage pregnant women have even greater nutrient needs to compensate for their continued growth as well as that of their unborn child.

The older population, especially women, also have special dietary needs. Lower energy needs limits this group to choosing foods from the four food groups only. However, care must be taken to get enough nutrients to meet nutrient needs, especially for calcium, folic acid, vitamin B12, riboflavin, and vitamins A and C. That's why it's important for this group to learn the value of nutrient density when making food choices.

One of the greatest values of the Guide to Good Eating is its outline of appropriate serving sizes from the Basic Four Food Group. Following the pattern would supply an adult wi th roughly 1,200 calories per day. Energy needs, however, vary with each individual, according to the USDA. The more energy you expend, the more you will need to consume. Vigorously active people, pregnant women, and children, especially teenagers, have high energy needs. Baseline nutrition must often be supplemented with energy-type foods—even a dip into the cookie jar. Making snacks nutritious as well as calorie-laden will assure adequate nutrient intake.

The Guide to Good Eating will be helpful in planning nutritionally adequate family meals. It will also help you control portion sizes if you follow the serving-size suggestions. These measures are especially valuable for people who are concerned about maintaining ideal weight to prevent overweight, as well as for those who want to reduce body weight.

GUIDE TO GOOD EATING

The recommended daily pattern provides the foundation for a nutritious, healthful diet.

The recommended servings from the Four Food Groups for adults supply about 1,200 calories. The chart below gives recommendations for the number and size of servings for several categories of people.

Food Group	Recommended Number of Servings				
	Child	Teenager	Adult	Pregnant Woman	Lactating Woman
Milk	3	4	2	4	4
1 cup milk, yogurt, OR **Calcium Equivalent:** 1½ slices (1½ oz.) Cheddar cheese* 1 cup pudding 1¾ cups ice cream 2 cups cottage cheese*					
Meat	2	2	2	3	2
2 ounces cooked, lean meat, fish, poultry, OR **Protein Equivalent:** 2 eggs 2 slices (2 oz. Cheddar cheese* ½ cup cottage cheese* 1 cup dried beans, peas 4 tbsp. peanut butter					
Fruit-Vegetable	4	4	4	4	4
½ cup cooked or juice 1 cup raw Portion commonly served such as a medium-size apple or banana					
Grain, whole grain, fortified, enriched 1 slice bread 1 cup ready-to-eat cereal ½ cup cooked cereal, pasta, grits	4	4	4	4	4

*Count cheese as serving of milk OR meat, not both simultaneously.

Foods in which fats and sugars are predominant complement but do not replace foods from the four food groups. Amounts have to be determined by individual caloric needs.

Courtesy of National Dairy Council, Rosemont, Illinois. ● 1977.

NUTRIENTS FOR HEALTH

Nutrients are chemical substances obtained from foods during digestion. They are needed to build and maintain body cells, regulate body processes, and supply energy.

About 50 nutrients, including water, are needed daily for optimum health. If one obtains the proper amount of the 10 "leader" nutrients in the daily diet, the other 40 or so nutrients will likely be consumed in amounts sufficient to meet body needs.

One's diet should include a variety of foods because no *single* food supplies all the 50 nutrients, and because many nutrients work together.

When a nutrient is added or a nutritional claim is made, nutrition labeling regulations require listing the 10 leader nutrients on food packages. These nutrients appear in the chart below with food sources and some major physiological functions.

Nutrient	Important Sources of Nutrient	
		Provide energy
Protein	Meat, Poultry, Fish Dried Beans and Peas Egg Cheese Milk	Supplies 4 calories per gram.
Carbohydrate	Cereal Potatoes Dried Beans Corn Bread Sugar	Supplies 4 calories per gram. Major source of energy for central nervous system.
Fat	Shortening, Oil Butter, Margarine Salad Dressing Sausages	Supplies 9 calories per gram.
Vitamin A (Retinol)	Liver Carrots Sweet Potatoes Greens Butter, Margarine	
Vitamin C (Ascorbic Acid)	Broccoli Orange Grapefruit Papaya Mango Strawberries	
Thiamin (B_1)	Lean Pork Nuts Fortified Cereal Products	Aids in utilization of energy.
Riboflavin (B_2)	Liver Milk Yogurt Cottage Cheese	Aids in utilization of energy.

Some major physiological functions

Build and maintain body cells

Constitutes part of the structure of every cell, such as muscle, blood, and bone; supports growth and maintains healthy body cells.

Supplies energy so protein can be used for growth and maintenance of body cells.

Constitutes part of the structure of every cell. Supplies essential fatty acids.

Assists formation and maintenance of skin and mucous membranes that line body cavities and tracts, such as nasal passages and intestinal tract, thus increasing resistance to infection.

Forms cementing substances, such as collagen, that hold body cells together, thus strengthening blood vessels, hastening healing of wounds and bones, and increasing resistance to infection.

Regulate body processes

Constitutes part of enzymes, some hormones and body fluids, and antibodies that increase resistance to infection.

Unrefined products supply fiber—complex carbohydrates in fruits, vegetables, and whole grains—for regular elimination.
Assists in fat utilization.

Provides and carries fat-soluble vitamins (A, D, E, and K).

Functions in visual processes and forms visual purple, thus promoting healthy eye tissues and eye adaptation in dim light.

Aids utilization of iron.

Functions as part of a coenzyme to promote the utilization of carbohydrate.
Promotes normal appetite.
Contributes to normal functioning of nervous system.

Functions as part of a coenzyme in the production of energy within body cells.
Promotes healthy skin, eyes, and clear vision.

Nutrient	Important Sources of Nutrient	Provide energy
Niacin	Liver Meat, Poultry, Fish Peanuts Fortified Cereal Products	Aids in utilization of energy.
Calcium	Milk, Yogurt Cheese Sardines and Salmon with Bones Collard, Kale, Mustard, and Turnip Greens	
Iron	Enriched Farina Prune Juice Liver Dried Beans and Peas Red Meat	Aids in utilization of energy.

Courtesy of National Dairy Council, Rosemont, Illinois. © 1977.

Some major physiological functions

Functions as part of a coenzyme in fat synthesis, tissue respiration, and utilization of carbohydrate. Promotes healthy skin, nerves, and digestive tract. Aids digestion and fosters normal appetite.

Combines with other minerals within a protein framework to give structure and strength to bones and teeth.

Assists in blood clotting.
Functions in normal muscle contraction and relaxation, and normal nerve transmission.

Combines with protein to form hemoglobin, the red substance in blood that carries oxygen to and carbon dioxide from the cells. Prevents nutritional anemia and its accompanying fatigue. Increases resistance to infection.

Functions as part of enzymes involved in tissue respiration.

Weight Control

Permit us this slight indulgence. We find it hard to disassociate good eating habits with proper weight control.

Of course, it's important for people to learn ways of lowering calories, but the calories we eat are so interlocked these days of massive overweight problems, we think a brief discussion on ways to control calories via weight control will help.

Elements other than calorie control are involved in this highly complex problem: life style consciousness, nutrient consciousness, portion control, eating habits, and exercise are some of the keys.

Life Style

Diet alone will not do the trick. People who have a life style concept of fitness and health often have little problem with weight control. They generally know how to control weight *before* it becomes a problem. We urge you to think in terms of developing a life style consciousness of sound eating habits, exercise, and fitness for best weight control.

Nutrients

Nutrient consciousness, as we have already pointed out, is more effective for controlling or losing weight than calorie consciousness. Nutrient consciousness is part of the total life style approach to health. Learning which foods provide ultimate nutrition will automatically limit calorie choices to those which give you something more than just fuel.

Portion Control

Portion control is another aspect of health consciousness and is easy to learn and adopt if you are hooked on fitness. The serving sizes provided in our recipes will teach you the value of portion control. You might also check the Guide to Good Eating recommendations (p. 257) to get an idea of what actually constitutes servings in each food group at different age levels. Little tricks, such as eating half the portion on your plate, can help you practice portion control, too. You won't have to count calories if you practice portion control.

Eating Habits

A change in life style eating habits comes with a change in life style consciousness. But some behavior modification techniques can be of value to help you "unlearn" poor eating habits. Here is a list of such techniques that have been developed over the past twenty years by various behaviorists:

• Establish one place in the house as your only dining spot. You'll restrict the opportunities to overeat.

• Eat slowly. Get into the habit of putting your fork down between bites. By establishing a slow eating pace you allow satiety to set in before too many calories have been consumed.

• Completely chew food before taking another biteful. The slower you eat, the less you will consume.

• Remove the serving dish from the table after everyone is served. Preferably, dish-up in the kitchen. Food out of sight is out of mind.

• Preplan your meals to avoid last-minute temptations to overeat.

• Avoid shopping when you are hungry.

• Keep snacking food out of the house. The less easily available, the less you will eat.

• Try to cut out at least one regularly consumed simple carbohydrate from your daily diet, such as a candy bar, cookie, or the sugar in your coffee.

• Consciously replace the urge to eat with an equally pleasing activity.

Exercise

We cannot stress enough the importance of consistent daily exercise for both weight control and overall fitness and well-being. We encourage you to adopt an exercise program, after consulting with your physician, that will suit your life style. Set realistic goals, starting an activity or exercise slowly at first, then building up gradually to a vigorous daily workout.

The benefits of exercise are many. Here are some gleaned from literature on exercise.

• Endurance-type activity, such as running, swimming, or brisk walking, are considered ideal for good cardiovascular health and weight control.

• Regular endurance-type exercise strengthens the heart muscles and increases the flow of blood to the heart. Studies now show that

active people have fewer heart attacks than inactive individuals.
- Exercise helps keep bones dense and retards bone loss as one ages.
- Exercise releases tension and acts as a natural tranquilizer.
- Exercise promotes a feeling of well-being and self-esteem.

Calculating Body Needs

There are many ways to calculate body needs for ideal weight maintenance.

The average individual needs at least 1,200 nutrient calories (not just calories) for proper baseline nutrition and weight control. Needs differ with individuals, however, depending on activity levels, body type, intensity of activity, or even inactivity.

Most individuals who lead moderately active lives need roughly 15 calories per pound of weight, which means that if your ideal body weight is 130 pounds you can eat up to 1,950 calories a day to maintain body weight. If, however, you are overweight, you will have to cut your calorie intake back and expend more energy to arrive at your ideal body weight. Since there are 3,500 calories in each pound of stored fat, you will need to consume 500 fewer calories each day until you arrive at your ideal weight.

Here is a formula that might be both fun and instructive in determining how you can maintain body weight.

Example:

    130 lb. (present weight)

    ×15 (calories activity level per pound weight)

    1,950 (calories needed to maintain present weight)

    −500 (calories daily to lose 1 pound per week*)

    1,450 (maximum daily calories needed to lose
           1 pound per week)

*For a two-pound weight loss per week, subtract 1,000 calories daily.

Activity versus Calories

Total calories expended per hour varies with the activity, one's body size, age, sex, and many other factors. This chart indicates *broadly* to what degree activity affects total calories used per hour.

Most charts vary slightly in numbers, so think of the chart as a broad-based guide rather than a true indication.

Activity	Calories Expended per Hour
Competitive swimming, running, and other vigorous, intense sports	600
Jogging, swimming, dancing, skating	350 to 450
Walking, bicycling, golf, housework	250 to 300
Light household chores, driving	120 to 180
Lying down, sitting	70 to 100

Nutrient Counter

The Nutrient Counter is your reference encyclopedia of food values. Restricted dieters will find it an invaluable table for comparing fat, sodium, calories, and cholesterol. It is also an excellent tool for recipe modification and will help you become a nutrient-wise shopper and meal planner. (Figures shown represent average nutrient values. These references include standard error of the mean.)

Adapted from: Charles Frederick Church and Helen Nichols Church, *Food Values of Portions Commonly Used* (Philadelphia: J. B. Lippincott, 1975); Barbara Kraus, *The Dictionary of Calories and Carbohydrates* (New York: Grosset & Dunlap, 1973); Barbara Kraus, *The Dictionary of Sodium, Fats, and Cholesterol* (New York: Grosset & Dunlap, 1974).

NUTRIENT COUNTER FOR COMMON FOODS

Food and Description	Measure or Quantity	Calories	Sodium mg	Cholesterol mg	Fat in Grams Total	Fat in Grams Saturated	Fat in Grams Unsaturated
A							
Alcohol (p. 280)							
Almonds, unsalted	6 almonds	48	tr	0	8.4	.1	8.3
Apple	1 medium	80	1	0	.8	--	--
Apple Juice, unsweetened	½ cup	58	1	0	tr	--	--
Apricot Jelly,							
low calorie	1 tablespoon	5	tr	0	tr	--	--
regular	1 tablespoon	54	5	0	tr	--	--
Arrowroot	1 tablespoon	29	tr	0	.2	--	--
Artichoke, fresh	1 medium	44	30	0	.4	--	--
Asparagus,							
fresh	5-6 spears	20	2	0	.1	--	--
Avocado	½ of 1 medium	185	4	--	18.4	--	--
B							
Baking Powder,							
low sodium	1 teaspoon	6	tr	0	tr	--	--
regular	1 teaspoon	6	276	0	tr	--	--
Baking Soda	1 teaspoon	neg	1000	0	0	--	--
Bamboo Shoots	½ cup	27	--	0	.4	--	--
Banana	1 medium	101	2	0	.2	--	--
Bean Sprouts	½ cup	16	3	0	tr	--	--
Beef (p. 276)							
Blackberries							
fresh	½ cup	41	tr	0	.7	--	--
frozen, unsweetened	4 oz.	54	1	0	.3	--	--
Blueberries,							
fresh	½ cup	45	1	0	.8	--	--
frozen, unsweetened	4 oz.	45	--	0	.6	--	--

Legend: tr = trace   neg = negligible   -- = figures unavailable

Food and Description	Measure or Quantity	Calories	Sodium mg	Cholesterol mg	Total	Saturated	Unsaturated
						Fat in Grams	
Bread							
rye	1 slice	70	128	0	.3	--	--
sourdough	1 slice	70	130	0	.7	--	--
white	1 slice	85	117	0	.7	--	--
whole wheat	1 slice	69	121	0	.6	--	--
Broccoli,							
fresh	½ cup	20	18	0	.2	--	--
frozen	½ cup	24	19	0	.8	--	--
Brown Sugar Substitute							
regular	1 tablespoon	neg	tr	0	--		
	1 tablespoon	48	tr	0	0		
Butter,							
salted	1 tablespoon	100	147	36	11.3	6	5
unsalted	1 tablespoon	100	1	35	11.3	6	5
C							
Cabbage, fresh	1 cup, shredded	22	18	0	.2	--	--
Cantaloupes, fresh	¼ of 5" melon	30	12	0	.1	--	--
Capers, bottled	1 tablespoon	6	306	0	0		
Carrots,							
fresh	1 large	21	24	0	.1	--	--
cooked	½ cup sliced	24	24	0	.2	--	--
Cashews, unsalted	6-8 nuts	84	21	0	4.9	.9	4
Catsup							
regular	1 tablespoon	18	263	0	tr	--	--
low sodium	1 tablespoon	19	4	0	tr	--	--
Cauliflower,							
raw	½ cup	14	6	.1	--	--	--
frozen	½ cup	16	9	0	.2	--	--
Celery							
fresh	1 cup, diced	20	134	0	--		
stalk	1 large	7	50	0	.2		
Cheese (p. 278)							
Chicken (p. 277)							
Chives, fresh	1 tablespoon	3	--	0	--		

Food	Serving						
Chocolate, semisweet	1 ounce (1 square)	132	4	0	9.2	--	--
chocolate chips	1 ounce	137	4	0	9.2	--	--
	½ cup	431	18	0	22	--	--
Cocoa	1 tablespoon	14	3	0	.7	--	--
chocolate wafer	1 wafer	20	29	0	.7	--	--
Coconut, shredded, unsweetened	1 tablespoon	42	1.21	0	3	--	--
Corn, fresh	1 ear	70	tr	0	1	--	--
frozen	½ cup	74	1	0	1	--	--
Cornmeal	1 cup	540	1	0	4.1	0	4.1
Cornstarch	1 tablespoon	29	--	0	tr	--	--
Cranberries, fresh	½ cup	23	1	0	.4	--	--
Cranberry Juice, unsweetened	½ cup	24	5	--	--	--	--
Cream Cheese	1 tablespoon	52	35	16	5.3	3.3	2
Crookneck Squash, fresh	½ cup	13	1	0	.2	--	--
frozen	½ cup	24	3	0	--	--	--
Cucumbers	1 medium	16	6	0	.2	--	--
E							
Egg Substitute*	1½ ounce	40	70	0	5.6	--	--
Egg, white only	1 medium	16	48	0	tr	--	--
Egg, whole	1 medium	80	53	220	5	2	3
Eggplant	½ cup	25	2	0	.2	--	--
Endive, Belgian	1 head	20	14	0	--	--	--
F							
Fettuccini Egg Noodles, cooked	½ cup	100	2	25	1.2	--	--
Fish (p. 276)							

*Nutrient count only for "Second Nature" egg substitute.

Legend: tr = trace   neg = negligible   -- = figures unavailable

Food and Description	Measure or Quantity	Calories	Sodium mg	Cholesterol mg	Fat in Grams Total	Saturated	Unsaturated
Flour,							
all-purpose	1 tablespoon	29	tr	0	.1	--	--
whole wheat	1 tablespoon	29	tr	0	.1	--	--
whole wheat or all-purpose	1 cup	414	2	0	1.2	--	--
Fructose	1 tablespoon	48	0	0	0	--	--
G							
Gelatin, unflavored	1 envelope	28	--	--	tr	--	--
Graham Cracker	1 cracker	30	41	tr	.7	tr	--
Grapefruit,							
fresh	½ medium	46	1	0	.1	--	--
canned, unsweetened	½ cup	45	1	0	.5	--	--
Grape Jelly, low calorie	1 tablespoon	15	tr	--	--	--	--
Grapes,							
fresh	20	54	2	0	.2	--	--
canned, unsweetened	½ cup	58	5	0	.1	--	--
Green Beans,							
fresh, cooked	½ cup	17	2	0	.1	--	--
frozen	½ cup	30	1	0	.1	--	--
Green Peppers	1 whole medium	31	8	--	.1	--	--
H							
Honey	1 tablespoon	61	1	0	0	--	--
Honeydew Melon	¼ of 5" melon	33	12	0	.3	--	--
Horseradish,							
dried	1 teaspoon	--	tr	0	tr	--	--
fresh	1 ounce	25	2	0	tr	--	--
prepared	1 ounce	3	312	0	tr	--	--
L							
Lamb (p. 276)							
Lasagna Noodles, cooked	½ cup	100	1.8	--	2.4	--	--
Leeks, trimmed (4 to 5)	4 ounces	59	6	0	.3	--	--
Lemon Juice	2 tablespoons	27	1	0	0	--	--

Food	Serving						
Lettuce,							
butter	¼ small head	14	9	0	.2	--	--
iceberg	¼ small head	14	9	0	.1	--	--
romaine	¼ small head	13	7	0	.2	--	--
Lima Beans,							
fresh, cooked	½ cup	94	--	0	.4	--	--
frozen, cooked	½ cup	131	--	0	.2	--	--
Liqueurs (p. 280)							
M							
Mandarin Oranges,							
canned, unsweetened	½ cup	31	2	0	tr	--	--
Maple Syrup,							
low-calorie	1 tablespoon	3	4	0	tr	--	--
regular	1 tablespoon	50	2	0	--	--	--
Margarine,							
low-calorie	1 tablespoon	50	110	0	5.6	1	5
regular	1 tablespoon	101	138	0	11.3	3	9
Marmalade,							
low-calorie	1 tablespoon	11	tr	0	0		
regular	1 tablespoon	60	tr	0	0		
Mayonnaise,							
low-sodium	1 tablespoon	85	1	0	9	--	--
low-calorie*	1 tablespoon	25	--	--	--	--	--
regular	1 tablespoon	101	84	10	11.2	2	9
Milk,							
buttermilk	1 cup	88	318	5	.2	--	--
evaporated nonfat	½ cup	96	165	2	.5	--	--
nonfat	1 cup	80	126	5	.2	--	--
whole	1 cup	159	122	34	8.5	5	3.5
low fat (2%)	1 cup	140	150	22	4.9	--	--

*Nutrient count is only for "Hollywood Imitation Mayonnaise."

Legend: tr = trace   neg = negligible   -- = figures unavailable

Food and Description	Measure or Quantity	Calories	Sodium mg	Cholesterol mg	Total	Saturated	Unsaturated
Mushrooms,							
fresh	½ cup	10	5	0	.1	--	--
canned	½ cup	21	488	0	.1	--	--
Mustard,							
dry	1 teaspoon	neg	1	0	tr	--	--
prepared	1 teaspoon	8	58	0	.4	--	--
Dijon	1 teaspoon	4	70	0	.2	--	--
N							
Noodles (egg), cooked	½ cup	100	1.5	25	2.4	.4	2
O							
Olive Oil	1 tablespoon	124	0	0	14	2	12
Onion,							
green	1 small	11	1	0	.1	--	--
Spanish, white	1 medium	38	10	0	.1	--	--
Orange	1 medium	77	2	0	.3	--	--
Orange Juice, unsweetened	½ cup	56	1	0	.2	--	--
Orange Marmalade,							
low-calorie	1 teaspoon	12	--	0	0		
regular	1 teaspoon	51	--	0	0		
P							
Papaya, fresh	½	44	4	0	.1	--	--
Pecans, unsalted	12 halves	96	tr	0	10	1	9
	½ cup chopped	357	tr	0	37		
Peaches,							
fresh	1 medium	38	1	0	.1	--	--
canned, unsweetened	½ cup	38	2	0	.1	--	--
Pea Pods, fresh	½ cup	58	2	0	.2	--	--
Pears,							
fresh	1 medium	90	3	0	.6	--	--
canned, unsweetened	½ cup	35	1	0	.2	--	--
Peas,							
fresh	½ cup	58	1	0	.3	--	--
frozen	½ cup	57	115	0	.3	--	--

Pimiento, canned, drained	¼ cup	15	18	0	.1	--	--
Pineapple Juice, unsweetened	½ cup	66	1	0	.1	--	--
Pineapple,							
fresh	1 slice	44	1	0	.2	--	--
canned, unsweetened	1 slice	33	.5	0	.5	--	--
crushed	½ cup	77	1	0	.1	--	--
Pistachio nuts, shelled	30 nuts	88	--	0	33.3	3	30
Pork (p. 276)							
Potato, Russet	1 medium	76	3	0	.1	--	--
sweet	1 medium	115	12	0	.5		
Poultry (p. 277)							
Pumpkin, canned, unsalted	½ cup	41	1	0	.1	--	--
R							
Radishes	2-3	7	7	0	.1	--	--
Raisins	1 tablespoon	29	3	0	.1	--	--
Raspberries,							
fresh	½ cup	41	--	0	.9	--	--
canned water-pack	½ cup	148	1	0	.2	--	--
Rice,							
brown, cooked	½ cup	135	--	0	.7	--	--
long grain, cooked	½ cup	87	--	0	.1	--	--
wild	½ cup	80	6	0	.6	--	--
S							
Safflower oil	1 tablespoon	124	0	0	14	1	13
Salt	1 teaspoon	0	2,325	0	0	--	--
Sesame Seeds	1 tablespoon	80	6	0	8	--	--
Sesame Seed Oil	1 tablespoon	124	0	0	5.1	--	--
Shallots	2 tablespoons, chopped	20	3	0	0	--	--
Shellfish (p. 277)							
Sour Cream,							
low-calorie	1 tablespoon	15	--	--	--	--	--
regular	1 tablespoon	28	6	8	4.5	--	--

Legend: tr = trace   neg = negligible   - - = figures unavailable

Food and Description	Measure or Quantity	Calories	Sodium mg	Cholesterol mg	Fat in Grams Total	Fat in Grams Saturated	Fat in Grams Unsaturated
Soy Sauce, regular	1 tablespoon	6	1,200	0	.2	--	--
Kikkoman Milder	1 tablespoon	10	605	0	0	--	--
Spaghetti, cooked	½ cup	100	2	--	2.4	.4	2
Spinach,							
fresh, raw	½ cup	8	12	0	.1	--	--
cooked	½ cup	18	19	0	.2		
frozen	½ cup	27	65	0	.3		
Squash,							
crookneck, fresh	½ cup	13	1	0	.2	--	--
zucchini, fresh	½ cup	9	1	0	.1	--	--
zucchini, frozen	½ cup	20	3	0	.1	--	--
winter	4 ounces	46	1	0	.1		
Strawberries,							
fresh	10	37	1	0	.7	--	--
frozen, unsweetened	4 ounces	25	1	0	.2	--	--
Sugar	1 tablespoon	48	0	0	0		
Sugar Substitutes							
Sucaryl	1 tablespoon	0	tr	0	0		
Sugar Twin	1 tablespoon	0	tr	0	0		
Sweet 'n Low	1 tablespoon	0	tr	0	0		
T							
Tartar Sauce	1 tablespoon	73	182	4	8	1	7
Tomatoes,							
fresh	1 medium	22	4	0	.3	--	--
low-sodium, canned	1 medium	25	3	0	.2	--	--
plum, fresh	1 medium	11	2	0	.2	--	--
Tomato Juice,							
regular, canned	½ cup	24	244	0	.1	--	--
low-sodium, canned	½ cup	20	3	0	.1	--	--
Tomato Purée,							
regular, canned	1 cup	97	998	0	.5	--	--
low-sodium, canned	1 cup	88	14	0	.5	--	--
Tomato Sauce, canned	1 cup	80	1,296	0	tr	--	--

Tortilla,						
corn	1 medium	42	..	0	.6	..	..
flour	1 medium	108	..	0	1.2	..	..
Turkey (p. 277)						
Turnips, fresh	½ cup	20	33	0	.1	..	..
V						
Vanilla Wafers	1 wafer	17	12	0	.7	..	..
Veal (p. 276)						
Vegetable Oil	1 tablespoon	124	0	0	14.2	2.2	12
V-8 Juice,						
regular, canned	½ cup	20	414	0	tr	..	..
low-sodium, canned	½ cup	20	16	0	tr	..	..
W						
Walnuts,						
chopped, raw, unsalted	½ cup	377	2	0	36.6	..	33
Water chestnuts, canned	4 ounces	90	23	0	.2	..	..
Watermelon	½ cup	26	1	0	1.5	..	..
Wines (p. 280)						
Worcestershire Sauce (French's)	1 tablespoon	6	150	tr	tr	..	..
Y						
Yams, fresh	½ cup	115	.2	0	..	..	..
Yogurt,						
fruit-flavored	1 cup	240	144	10	3.2	2	1
plain, made from partially skimmed milk	1 cup	122	116	18	3.9	2	2
Plain, made from whole milk	1 cup	151	115	30	8.2	4	4
Z						
Zwieback Crackers	1 piece	31	6	0	.7	..	..

Legend: tr = trace   neg = negligible   .. = figures unavailable

Nutrient Counter   275

NUTRIENT COUNTER FOR MEATS

Meat	Calories	Sodium mg	Cholesterol mg	Total Fat g
BEEF				
Chuck				
Blade Roast	263	56	83	13
Arm Pot Roast	263	56	83	13
Ground Beef, lean (80%)	263	56	83	17
Rib				
Rib Roast Small End	285	56	83	6
Rib Steak	262	56	83	17
Loin				
Sirloin Steak	208	56	83	11
Porterhouse Steak	242	56	83	15
Tenderloin Steak	224	56	83	13
T-bone Steak	247	56	83	15
Flank				
Flank Steak	235	56	83	10
Round				
Rump Roast	235	56	83	11
Top Round Steak	229	56	83	5
Bottom Round Steak	238	56	83	9
Tip Roast	186	56	83	7
Beef Stew (round)	260	56	83	14
Ground Beef, lean (90%)	163	56	83	4
VEAL				
Rib Chop	215	75	96	8
Loin Chop	207	75	96	7
Rump Roast	175	75	96	5
Veal Cutlet	202	75	96	6
PORK				
Shoulder				
Arm Picnic	246	60	82	15
Loin				
Sirloin Roast, lean only	227	60	82	11
Loin Chops, lean only	250	60	82	11
Tenderloin, lean only	255	60	82	12
Smoked Ham				
Whole	219	1,012	56	9.24
LAMB				
Shoulder				
Blade Chop	280	66	92	18
Rib Chop	290	66	92	20
Loin Chop	223	66	92	12
Leg Whole	195	66	92	8
FISH				
Codfish	78	70	50	tr
Haddock	79	61	70	tr
Halibut	100	54	36	1
Mackerel (Pacific)	191	- -	86	7

Courtesy of the United States Department of Agriculture, *Composition of Foods*, Agricultural Handbook No. 8, 1963.

Meat	Calories	Sodium mg	Cholesterol mg	Total Fat g
FISH (continued)				
Perch	118	77	70	4
Pike	93	51	78	1
Red Snapper	89	63	63	tr
Salmon	119	64	54	4
Sole	73	73	60	7
Swordfish	106	--	83	3
Trout	195	20	63	11
Tuna,				
unsalted water-pack	127	41	56	1
salted, canned in oil	288	800	56	21
SHELLFISH				
Abalone	89	--	72	.2
Clams	82	102	47	2
Crab	93	--	93	2
Lobster	91	210	79	2
Oyster	66	73	50	2
Scallops	76	255	33	tr
Shrimp	91	140	141	.9
POULTRY				
Chicken, dark meat				
(no skin)	112	83	59	3.3
(with skin)	177	63	82	5.6
Chicken, light meat				
(no skin)	101	83	59	1.3
(with skin)	154	46	63	3.3
Turkey, dark meat				
(no skin)	120	92	95	7
(with skin)	200	122	109	17
Turkey, light meat				
(no skin)	109	77	72	1.7
(with skin)	189	47	86	12

NOTE: All quantities are 3.5 ounce servings (100 grams).

NUTRIENT COUNTER FOR CHEESES

Note: All quantities are 1 ounce unless otherwise indicated.

Cheese	Calories	Sodium mg	Cholesterol mg	Fat in Grams		
				Total	Saturated	Unsaturated
Blue	100	396	21	8.15	5.30	2.85
Brick	105	159	27	8.41	5.32	3.09
Brie	95	178	28	7.85	--	--
Camembert	85	239	20	6.88	4.33	2.55
Cheddar	114	176	30	9.40	5.98	3.42
Colby	112	171	27	9.10	5.73	3.37
Cottage, creamed (1 cup)	217	850	31	9.47	5.99	3.48
Cottage, 2% low fat (1 cup)	203	918	19	4.36	2.76	1.60
Cottage, 1% low fat (1 cup)	164	918	10	2.30	1.46	.84
Cottage, dry curd (1 cup)	123	19	10	.61	.40	.21
Cream Cheese	99	84	31	9.89	6.23	3.66
Edam	101	274	25	7.88	4.98	2.90
Feta	75	316	25	6.03	4.24	1.79
Gouda	101	232	32	7.78	4.99	2.79
Gruyère	117	95	31	9.17	5.36	3.81
Limburger	93	227	26	7.72	4.75	2.97
Monterey Jack	106	152	--	8.58	--	--
Mozzarella, part skim	80	106	22	6.12	3.73	2.39
Muenster	104	178	27	8.52	5.42	3.10
Parmesan, grated	129	528	22	8.51	5.41	3.10
grated (1 tablespoon)	31	88	--	1.7	--	--
Provolone	100	248	20	7.55	4.82	2.73
Ricotta, whole milk (1 cup)	428	207	124	31.93	20.41	11.52
Ricotta, part skim milk (1 cup)	340	307	76	19.46	12.12	7.34
Romano	110	340	29	7.64	--	--
Swiss	107	74	26	7.78	5.04	2.74

Cheese	Calories	Sodium mg	Cholesterol mg	Fat in Grams		
				Total	Saturated	Unsaturated
Pasteurized Process						
American	106	406	27	8.86	5.58	3.28
Swiss	95	388	24	7.09	4.55	2.54
Swiss Cheese Food	92	440	23	6.84	--	--
American Cheese Spread	82	381	16	6.02	3.78	2.24
Low-Sodium Cheeses						
American	110	10	--	9	--	--
Gouda	110	10	--	9	--	--

Courtesy of the United States Department of Agriculture, *Composition of Foods*, Agricultural Handbook No. 8, 1963.

Alcohol Exchange List

Everyone should be aware of alcohol's effect on the body. Alcohol is not only high in calories (about 140 calories per 2 ounces), but it also tends to lower the sugar levels in the blood rather than elevate them. Diabetics and hypoglycemics who must avoid rises in insulin must control their intake of alcoholic beverages and should be advised by their physicians or dietitians on their use.

The Alcohol Exchange List is designed to help plan alcohol intake carefully. It lists the alcoholic calories of commonly consumed alcoholic beverages in normal servings with appropriate bread and fat exchanges.

ALCOHOL EXCHANGE

Beverages	Amount	Calories	Exchange
Distilled			
Gin, Rum, Vodka, Whiskey	1 ounce	70	2 fat exchanges
Brandy	1 ounce	73	1 bread exchange
Cognac	1 ounce	73	1 bread exchange
Liqueurs			
Cordial-Anisette	1½ ounces	74	1 bread exchange
Apricot Brandy	1 ounce	86	1 bread exchange
Benedictine	1 ounce	112	1 bread exchange
Crème de Menthe	1 ounce	94	1 bread exchange
Curaçao	1½ ounces	84	1 bread exchange
Wine			
Port	3½ ounces	84	1 bread exchange ½ fat exchange
Dry Sherry	2 ounces	84	⅓ bread exchange 1½ fat exchanges
Champagne, extra dry	3 ounces	87	½ bread exchange 1 fat exchange
Dubonnet	3 ounces	96	½ bread exchange 1½ fat exchanges
Madeira	3 ounces	120	1 bread, 1 fat
Dry Marsala	3 ounces	124	2 bread exchanges 2 fat exchanges
Sweet Marsala	3 ounces	182	2 bread exchanges ½ fat exchange
Muscatel	4 ounces	158	1 bread exchange 2 fat exchanges
Dry Red Wine	3 ounces	64	1 bread exchange
Sake	3 ounces	75	½ bread exchange ½ fat exchange
Dry Vermouth	3½ ounces	112	1½ bread exchanges
Sweet Vermouth	3½ ounces	151	1½ bread exchanges ½ fat exchange
Dry White Wine	3 ounces	74	1 bread exchange
Beer	12 ounces	151	1 bread exchange 2 fat exchanges

Spices and Herbs

Feel free to experiment with your own herb and spice concoctions. The adventure will be well worth the effort. You'll see after working with our recipes how effective spices and herbs can be. And fun, too.

Start with a small amount and gradually build up to amounts desired. Be careful with the overpowering spices, such as cloves, nutmeg, cardamom, anise, mace, saffron, and ginger. A little goes a long way. You can be generous with such herbs as parsley, garlic, basil, oregano, and rosemary, especially when they're used fresh. Fresh herbs impart true flavors and are ideal in salads and sauces. A judicious touch of pepper can perk up a saltless soup or stock. Too much can ruin it. Caraway or other seeds are good flavor additions to breads, dressings, and baked goods. Here are some tips from USDA consumer advisors, as well as those based on our experiences with herbs and spices.

As a general rule, herbs and spices should be added toward the end of cooking, as flavor of ground spices is imparted immediately. The flavor of fresh herbs takes longer to release so they are added early in cooking. Whole spices are best in slow cooking and could be tied in cheesecloth bags for steeping in sauces and soups. Toasting seeds enhances their aroma and flavor. Whole dried leaves impart superior flavor when ground or pulverized just before adding to foods.

It's best to purchase small amounts at a time, as spices and herbs tend to lose their flavor and color during long storage. Store them in a cool, dry place in airtight containers. A warm spot may hasten flavor deterioration, and damp environments cause caking and infestation. Spices will retain maximum aroma and flavor up to six months of storage. Herbs tend to lose flavor more rapidly than ground ginger, pepper, cinnamon, and cloves. Pick off bruised leaves and discard stems for they tend to cause bitterness.

It's best to replenish your supply of herbs and spices at least once every six to eight months to give your cooked foods the best flavor chance possible.

You might even decide to pot your own herbs for year-round supplies at your fingertips. And so much less expensive, too.

And Wines, Too

The *Light Style* approach to cooking relies heavily on ways of improving the flavor of foods cooked without salt. The effective use of herbs and spices is one way to beat the flavor blues. Wines are another.

Light Style treats wine as a seasoning. And as a seasoning, a little goes a long way. After all, we want to bring out, not mask, flavors.

A few words about cooking with spirits. Heat causes alcohol to evaporate, leaving only the residue of flavor and sugar calories if present. There are negligible calories when spirits are used in small amounts. There are 64 calories in 3 ounces of red wine, or 11 calories per tablespoon. If you are on a sodium-restricted diet, avoid so-called "cooking wines," as they are higher in sodium than regular wines.

A touch of wine can add flavor to fish or fowl. It can bring out the rich flavor of sauces, stews, or soups and serve as a natural tenderizer for meats when used as a marinade. It does wonders to bring out flavor of meat when used as a basting sauce.

Wines used in sweet dishes and fruit should be treated much like vanilla. A small amount will do the trick. It's best to allow flavors to meld when combining wines with fruit. Wine is usually the last ingredient added to sauces, soups, or stews, however.

Although there is no hard and fast rule about using red or white wine, a general rule of thumb is to use white wine with light foods (vegetables, fish, or fowl) and red wines with red meats.

Uses of Spices and Herbs

Spice	Uses
Allspice	Pot roast, fish, eggs, pickles, sweet potatoes, squash, fruit.
Anise Seed	Cookies, cakes, breads, candy, cheese, beverages, pickles, beef stew, stewed fruits, fish.
Basil	Tomatoes, noodles, rice, beef stew, pork, meat loaf, duck, fish, veal, green or vegetable salad, eggplant, potatoes, carrots, spinach, peas, eggs, cheese, jelly.
Bay Leaf	Soups, chowders, pickles, fish, pot roast, variety meats, stews, marinades.

Caraway Seed	Green beans, beets, cabbage, carrots, cauliflower, potatoes, sauerkraut, turnips, zucchini, goose, lamb, pork, spareribs, beef or lamb stew, marinades for meats, cake, cookies, rice, rye bread.
Cardamom	Baked goods, pickles, grape jelly, puddings, sweet potatoes, squash, fruit soups.
Cayenne Pepper	Meat dishes, spaghetti, pizza, chicken, fish, eggs, cheese, vegetables, pickles.
Celery Seed	Potato salad, fruit salad, tomatoes, vegetables, stuffings, pickles, breads, rolls, egg dishes, meat loaf, stews, soups. Celery powder may be used in any of the above.
Chili Powder	Tomato or barbecue sauces, dips, egg dishes, stews, meat loaf, chicken, marinades for meats, cheese, bean casseroles, corn, eggplant.
Cinnamon	Beverages, bakery products, fruits, pickles, pork, ham, lamb or beef stews, roast lamb, chicken.
Cloves	Fruits, pickles, baked goods, fish, stuffings, meat sauces, pot roast, marinades for meats, green beans, Harvard beets, carrots, sweet potatoes, tomatoes. Used whole to stud ham, fruit, glazed pork, beef.
Curry Powder	Curried beef, chicken, fish, lamb, meatballs, pork, veal, eggs, dried beans, fruit, dips, breads, marinades for meats.
Dill Seed	Pickles, pickled beets, salads, sauerkraut, green beans, egg dishes, stews, fish, chicken, breads.
Fennel Seed	Egg dishes, fish, stews, marinades for meats, vegetables, cheese, baked or stewed apples, pickles, sauerkraut, breads, cakes, cookies.
Garlic	Tomato dishes, soups, dips, sauces, salads, salad dressings, dill pickles, meat, poultry, fish stews, marinades, bread.

Spices and Herbs 283

Ginger	Pickles, conserves, baked or stewed fruits, vegetables, baked products, beef, lamb, pork, veal, poultry, fish, beverages, soups, oriental dishes.
Mace	Baked products, fruits, meat loaf, fish, poultry, chowder, vegetables, jellies, pickles, breads.
Marjoram	Lamb, pork, beef, veal, chicken, fish, tomato dishes, carrots, cauliflower, peas, spinach, squash, mushrooms, broccoli, pizza, spaghetti, egg dishes, breads, soups.
Mint	Punches, tea, sauces for desserts, sauces for lamb, mint jelly, sherbet, vegetables, lamb stew, lamb roast.
Dry Mustard	Egg and cheese dishes, salad dressings, meat, poultry, vegetables.
Mustard Seed	Cucumber pickles, corned beef, coleslaw, potato salad, boiled cabbage, sauerkraut.
Nutmeg	Hot beverages, puddings, baked products, fruits, chicken, seafood, eggs, vegetables, pickles, conserves.
Onion Powder	Dips, soups, stews, all meats, fish, poultry, salads, vegetables, stuffing, cheese dishes, egg dishes, breads, rice dishes.
Oregano	Tomatoes, pasta sauces, pizza, chili con carne, barbecue sauce, vegetable soup, egg and cheese dishes, onions, stuffings, pork, lamb, chicken, fish.
Paprika	Beef, pork, veal, lamb, sausage, game, fish, poultry, egg dishes, cheese dishes, vegetables lacking color, pickles.
Parsley	Soups, coleslaw, breads, tomato and meat sauces, stuffings, broiled or fried fish, meats, poultry.
Pepper: Black	Meats, poultry, fish, eggs, vegetables, pickles.

Cayenne	Meats, soups, cheese dishes, sauces, pickles, poultry, vegetables, spaghetti sauce, curried dishes, dips, tamale pie, barbecued beef and pork.
White	White or light meats, vegetables.
Poppy Seed	Pie crust, scrambled eggs, fruit compotes, cheese sticks, fruit salad dressings, cookies, cakes, breads, noodles. Sprinkle over top of fruit salads, vegetables, breads, cookies and cakes.
Poultry Seasoning	Stuffings, poultry, veal, meat loaf, chicken soup.
Rosemary	Lamb, poultry, veal, beef. pork, fish, soups, stews, marinades, potatoes, cauliflower, spinach, mushrooms, turnips, fruits, breads.
Saffron	Baked goods, chicken, seafood, rice, curries.
Sage	Stuffings for poultry, fish, and other meats, sauces, soups, chowders, poultry, fish, beef, pork, veal, marinades, lima beans, onions, eggplant, tomatoes, cheese, potatoes.
Sesame Seed	Sprinkle on canapes, breads, cookies, casseroles, salads, noodles, soups, vegetables. Add to pie crust, pie fillings, cakes, cookies, dips, stuffings.
Tarragon	Sour cream sauces, casseroles, marinades, pot roasts, veal, lamb, poultry, fish, egg dishes.
Thyme	Meat, poultry, fish, vegetables.
Turmeric	Cakes, breads, curried meats, fish, poultry, egg dishes, rice dishes, pickles.
Vanilla	Baked goods, beverages, puddings.

Adapted from The United States Department of Agriculture Research Service, Consumer and Food Economics Institute.

Table of Substitutions

The Table of Substitutions is your tool for modifying recipes accurately. It contains the conversions for regular and artificial sweeteners according to brand, herbs and spices, as well as a wide variety of other commonly used ingredients necessary for even the strictest dietary modification.

Although we do not encourage the use of artificial sweeteners, we have listed them for those who are medically advised to do so. Generally speaking, a small amount of the sweeteners may not be harmful. If you drink large quantities of liquid sweetened with them, however, you may wish to reconsider its use. As of this writing, the Food and Drug Administration ruling on saccharin states that additional research is needed to determine whether saccharin is safe for use. The FDA warns, however, that saccharin may cause cancer, and a sign to this effect must be conspicuously posted in stores wherever saccharin is used by the consumer and food industry. The American Diabetes Association does, however, advocate the use of saccharin for diabetics.

We have included the Table of Substitutions for fructose, the natural fruit sugar available in crystalline and liquid form. The calorie-lowering effect could be worth the expense if you use it frequently. The caloric saving when used in small amounts may not be worth the bother, much less the expense. Fructose has no specific government regulatory limitations, and is considered safe as a nutritive sweetener, but the word is moderation as with table sugar. Those who use sizable quantities of it may wish to consider its use as a calorie-lowering sweetener.

Fructose and sugar contain exactly the same caloric value—48 calories per tablespoon. Because fructose is 1½ times sweeter than sugar, however, only half as much is needed for sweetening. You would use ½ teaspoon fructose in lieu of 1 teaspoon sugar.

Fructose tends to enhance the flavor of foods cooked without salt. It is, in fact, a high-potency flavoring agent, like salt, but in a sweet form. It's also a good sweetener for mixing in beverages. Fructose also has a dental health advantage because less is needed to produce sweetness in candies, gums, and other foods associated with dental caries.

Salt is America's most overworked seasoning. The total daily salt intake of 8 grams recommended by the U.S. Senate Committee on Dietary Goals has little chance. A mere "salting to taste" at the table can add 800 milligrams without really trying. It would seem wise for high salters to learn ways of substituting or cutting salt down or out. Substituting herbs, spices, wines, and juices will help do just that!

Arrowroot and cornstarch substitutes for flour follow the principle of using less for fewer calories because the thickening effect is greater than that of flour. You'll get the thickening effect and a shinier, smoother texture for half the calories of flour.

We do not necessarily endorse commercial egg substitute. We give it as an ingredient in our recipes only as an example to show how calories can be cut to a maximum degree or how cholesterol can be reduced if medically necessary.

Table of Equivalents

Item		Substitution

Artificial Sweeteners (Sugar Substitutes)

Sugar Twin:
 1 teaspoon = 1 teaspoon sugar

Sugar Twin, Brown:
 1 teaspoon = 1 teaspoon sugar

Sweet 'N Low:
 ¹⁄₁₀ teaspoon = 1 teaspoon sugar
 ⅓ teaspoon = 1 tablespoon sugar
 1 teaspoon = ⅙ cup sugar
 1½ teaspoons = ¼ cup sugar
 3 teaspoons = ½ cup sugar
 6 teaspoons (2 tablespoons) = 1 cup sugar

Adolph's Sugar Substitute:
 2 shakes of jar = 1 rounded teaspoon sugar
 ¼ teaspoon = 1 tablespoon sugar
 1 teaspoon = ¼ cup sugar
 2½ teaspoons = ⅔ cup sugar
 1 tablespoon = ¾ cup sugar
 4 teaspoons = 1 cup sugar

Sucaryl (Liquid Sweetener):
 ⅛ teaspoon = 1 teaspoon sugar
 ½ teaspoon = 4 teaspoons sugar
 ¾ teaspoon = 2 tablespoons sugar
 1½ teaspoons = ¼ cup sugar
 3 teaspoons (1 tablespoon) = ½ cup sugar

Fructose
 ½ teaspoon = 1 teaspoon sugar
 1½ teaspoons = 1 tablespoon sugar
 2 tablespoons = ¼ cup sugar
 ¼ cup fructose = ½ cup sugar
 6 tablespoons = ¾ cups sugar
 ½ cup = 1 cup sugar

Item		Substitution

Herbs, Spices, Seasonings:

Garlic Powder:
⅛ teaspoon = 1 small clove garlic

Ginger, Powdered
½ teaspoon = 1 teaspoon, fresh

Herbs, Dried:
1 teaspoon = 1 tablespoon, fresh

Horseradish, fresh:
1 tablespoon = 2 tablespoons, bottled

Miscellaneous:

Baking Powder:
1 teaspoon = 1 teaspoon baking soda +
½ teaspoon cream of tartar

  Low-Sodium:
1½ teaspoon = ½ teaspoon baking powder

Chocolate:
1 square (1 ounce) = 3 tablespoons cocoa +
1 tablespoon shortening

Gelatin, powdered:
1 envelope (¼ ounce) = 1 tablespoon

Yeast, Active Dry:
1 envelope = ¾ tablespoon to be reconstituted in 2 tablespoons
water

Low-Sodium Baking Powder:
  Your druggist can make it for you by using the
following formula. (This formula yields about 4½ ounces.)

Potassium bicarbonate	39.8 grams
Cornstarch	20.0 grams
Tartaric acid	7.5 grams
Potassium bitartrate	56.1 grams

Arrowroot:
  1½ teaspoons arrowroot for 1 tablespoon flour
  ⅔ tablespoon arrowroot for 1 tablespoon cornstarch

Table of Measurement Equivalents

Comparison of Avoirdupois and Metric Units of Weight

1 oz = 0.06 lb = 28.35 g   1 lb = 0.454 kg
2 oz = 0.12 lb = 56.70 g   2 lb = 0.91 kg
3 oz = 0.19 lb = 85.05 g   3 lb = 1.36 kg
4 oz = 0.25 lb = 113.40 g   4 lb = 1.81 kg
5 oz = 0.31 lb = 141.75 g   5 lb = 2.27 kg
6 oz = 0.38 lb = 170.10 g   6 lb = 2.72 kg
7 oz = 0.44 lb = 198.45 g   7 lb = 3.18 kg
8 oz = 0.50 lb = 226.80 g   8 lb = 3.63 kg
9 oz = 0.56 lb = 255.15 g   9 lb = 4.08 kg
10 oz = 0.62 lb = 283.50 g   10 lb = 4.54 kg
11 oz = 0.69 lb = 311.85 g
12 oz = 0.75 lb = 340.20 g
13 oz = 0.81 lb = 368.55 g
14 oz = 0.88 lb = 396.90 g
15 oz = 0.94 lb = 425.25 g
16 oz = 1.00 lb = 453.59 g

1 g = 0.035 oz   1 kg = 2.205 lb
2 g = 0.07 oz   2 kg = 4.41 lb
3 g = 0.11 oz   3 kg = 6.61 lb
4 g = 0.14 oz   4 kg = 8.82 lb
5 g = 0.18 oz   5 kg = 11.02 lb
6 g = 0.21 oz   6 kg = 13.23 lb
7 g = 0.25 oz   7 kg = 15.43 lb
8 g = 0.28 oz   8 kg = 17.64 lb
9 g = 0.32 oz   9 kg = 19.84 lb
10 g = 0.35 oz   10 kg = 22.05 lb

Adapted from "Handbook of Food Preparation," American Home Economics Association, © 1975.

Comparison of U.S. and Metric Units of Liquid Measure

1 fl oz = 29.573 ml	1 qt = 0.946 l	1 gal = 3.785 l
2 fl oz = 59.15 ml	2 qt = 1.89 l	2 gal = 7.57 l
3 fl oz = 88.72 ml	3 qt = 2.84 l	3 gal = 11.36 l
4 fl oz = 118.30 ml	4 qt = 3.79 l	4 gal = 15.14 l
5 fl oz = 147.87 ml		
6 fl oz = 177.44 ml		
7 fl oz = 207.02 ml		
8 fl oz = 236.59 ml		
9 fl oz = 266.16 ml		
10 fl oz = 295.73 ml		

1 ml = 0.034 fl oz	1 l = 1.057 qt	1 l = 0.264 gal
2 ml = 0.07 fl oz	2 l = 2.11 qt	2 l = 0.53 gal
3 ml = 0.10 fl oz	3 l = 3.17 qt	3 l = 0.79 gal
4 ml = 0.14 fl oz	4 l = 4.23 qt	4 l = 1.06 gal
5 ml = 0.17 fl oz	5 l = 5.28 qt	5 l = 1.32 gal
6 ml = 0.20 fl oz.	6 l = 6.34 qt	6 l = 1.59 gal
7 ml = 0.24 fl oz	7 l = 7.40 qt	7 l = 1.85 gal
8 ml = 0.27 fl oz	8 l = 8.45 qt	8 l = 2.11 gal
9 ml = 0.30 fl oz	9 l = 9.51 qt	9 l = 2.38 gal
10 ml = 0.34 fl oz	10 l = 10.57 qt	10 l = 2.64 gal

Equivalents for One Unit and Fractions of a Unit

Tablespoon
1 Tbsp = 3 tsp
¾ Tbsp = 2¼ tsp
⅔ Tbsp = 2 tsp
½ Tbsp = 1½ tsp
⅓ Tbsp = 1 tsp
¼ Tbsp = ¾ tsp

Cup
1 c = 16 Tbsp
¾ c = 12 Tbsp
⅔ c = 10⅔ Tbsp
½ c = 8 Tbsp
⅓ c = 5⅓ Tbsp
¼ c = 4 Tbsp
⅛ c = 2 Tbsp
1/16 c = 1 Tbsp

Pint
1 pt = 2 c
¾ pt = 1½ c
⅔ pt = 1⅓ c
½ pt = 1 c
⅓ pt = ⅔ c
¼ pt = ½ c
⅛ pt = ¼ c
1/16 pt = 2 Tbsp

Quart
1 qt = 2 pt
¾ qt = 3 c
⅔ qt = 2⅔ c
½ qt = 1 pt
⅓ qt = 1⅓ c
¼ qt = 1 c
⅛ qt = ½ c
1/16 qt = ¼ c

Gallon
1 gal = 4 qt
¾ gal = 3 qt

½ gal = 2 qt
⅓ gal = 5⅓ c
¼ gal = 1 qt
⅛ gal = 1 pt
1/16 gal = 1 c

Pound
1 lb = 16 oz
¾ lb = 12 oz
⅔ lb = 10⅔ oz
½ lb = 8 oz
⅓ lb = 5⅓ oz
¼ lb = 4 oz
⅛ lb = 2 oz
1/16 lb = 1 oz

Meat Thermometer

A meat thermometer is the best inexpensive gadget investment any cook can make. It will tell you when roasted beef is just medium rare and when poultry is done before it becomes too dry. Stick the thermometer in the thickest part of a roast or the breast of poultry away from any bone. Cook the meat until the thermometer reaches the desired degree of doneness, as indicated on the following charts. Ideally, however, remove the meat from the oven when the internal temperature is 5 to 10 degrees below the temperature at which the meat is to be served to avoid overcooking. Roasted meats continue to cook after removal from the oven.

Degree of doneness of any meat is a highly personal matter. Such meats as pork do, however, require long, complete cooking to kill any harmful bacteria or parasites (trichina, a parasitic worm). While you must have high temperature readings for pork, you may have a personal preference when it comes to lamb. Middle Easterners like their lamb falling into shreds from overcooking, while the American prefers a rather rosy pink lamb chop or roast. The choice is yours. Poultry should be succulent at 180°F, depending on the bird, its age and species. The longer a game bird cooks, the more tender and succulent it will be. Turkey is an exception. Turkeys are, these days, grown for tender meat. The proper temperature would depend on the bird, but a safe rule-of-thumb is to remove it from the oven when the thermometer hits 175 to 180°F. Even more touchy is the question of roast beef. If you get thermometer readings below 130°F you're in sub-rare territory, reserved for afficionados of blood-red meat.

Reserve the thermometer for oven roasting only, but do use it. It will be your best indicator of doneness.

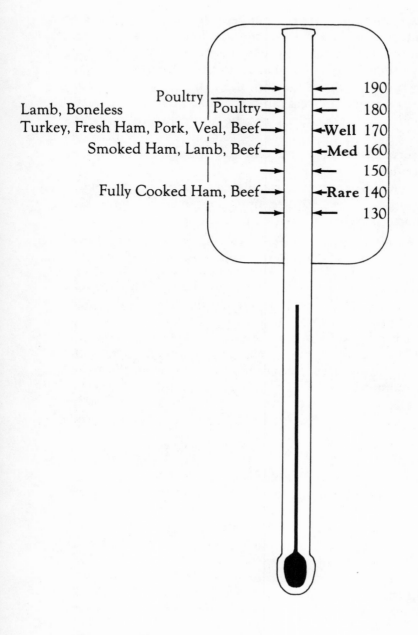

Poultry

Lamb, Boneless
Turkey, Fresh Ham, Pork, Veal, Beef→
Smoked Ham, Lamb, Beef→

Fully Cooked Ham, Beef→

Poultry→

←190
←180
←Well 170
←Med 160
←150
←Rare 140
←130

Specialty Products

The products listed here are brands which we have found to be the lowest in sodium, fat, and calories and, in our opinion, highest in flavor over all others. This list is not, however, an endorsement of these products, but a practical solution for those who must use them when medical needs dictate it. In fact, we strongly advise the use of natural ingredients whenever possible.

Because supermarket inventories differ markedly from region to region and may or may not include the product you are looking for, we suggest you call before you dash off to the market. Ask the store manager to order the product if he does not carry it. If he won't, you may want to write to the food company for a source in your area. You might also check with your local hospital dietitian for sources or refer to the list of some of the major suppliers on p. 296.

Label information on products can be a great help in describing and analyzing the product before you decide to buy it. With the exception of certain products, the Food and Drug Administration requires that labels provide minimum information, such as how much the contents weigh, the name of the manufacturer and/or distributor, and a description of the product. Ingredients are listed in descending order of amount, with the top five indicating largest amounts. If the label, for instance, lists fat, sugar, or salt as the first ingredient, you will know that that ingredient predominates.

The Food and Drug Administration ruling effective 1 July 1979 requires that foods labeled as "low calorie" must contain no more than 40 calories per serving; foods labeled "reduced calories" will have to be at least one-third lower than their counterparts; and if the product is labeled "reduced calories," it must state the number of calories contained in the comparable food.

Here are a few general comments about some of the listings that follow.

+ Low-sodium products are suggested especially for those on salt-restricted diets. Most canned foods contain high levels of salt, so check all packaged food labels for salt content.

+ Fructose, the natural fruit sugar found in all plants, fruits and berries, is 50 percent of the dry substance of honey and is a constituent of sugar. Fructose behaves much like sugar. It is water soluble, but also the sweetest of all commonly found sugars (it's about 1½ times sweeter than sucrose, ordinary table sugar). Because of its excessive sweetness, less is used. The total calories, therefore, are reduced as well. Its high cost of production, however, keeps fructose a high-priced sweetener. Consumers should weigh the calorie-lowering advantages against the high cost.

Another health benefit is its possible value for diabetics and hypoglycemics, since it needs no insulin to be absorbed. Fructose is still a sugar, however, and has carbohydrate calories that must be accounted for in a diabetic diet. Diabetics should consult their physician or dietitian for advice on its use. The amounts used in our recipes should pose no problems for diet-controlled diabetics. The diabetic exchange information included in the nutrient analysis for each recipe will also help make proper adjustments.

• Low-calorie toppings have no specific food value, but we have listed them for those who must restrict fat intake. Another idea is to make your own using our recipe, Heavenly Whipped Topping (p. 205).

Sources for Special Products

Jolly Jon Products
Ener-G Foods
1526 Utah Avenue
South Seattle, Washington 98134

Fisher Cheeses
Fisher Cheese Co.
Department THTO
Box 409
Wapakonet, Ohio 45895

General Mills Products
General Mills Chemical Corp.
Dietetic Specialties
4620 West 77th Street
Minneapolis, Minnesota 55435

Product	Brand Name	Where Distributed	Comments
CHEESES			
Low-sodium Cheddar cheese	Tillamook, Schreibers	Health food stores	
Cheez-Ola Count Down	Fisher Cheeses	Most supermarkets and health food stores	
Low-fat cottage cheese	Knudsen	Supermarkets	
Low-fat, low-sodium cottage cheese	Edgemar Farms	Supermarkets	
Low-sodium Gouda		Hickory Farms	
Hoop cheese	Knudsen	Supermarkets	
CONDIMENTS, etc.			
Low-sodium baking powder	Cellu	Supermarkets and health food stores	
Low-sodium catsup	Cellu, Tillie Lewis Tasti Diet	Supermarkets and health food stores	Good flavor.
Low-sodium chili sauce	Cellu	Health food stores and some supermarkets	
Low-calorie jelly	Smuckers	Supermarkets	Good flavor.
Low-sodium, low-calorie mayonnaise	Hollywood	Supermarkets and health food stores	
Low-calorie mayonnaise	Tillie Lewis Tasti Diet	Supermarkets and health food stores	Contains approximately one-fourth the calories of regular mayonnaise.
Mayonnaise, imitation	Kraft	Supermarkets and health food stores	

Product	Brand Name	Where Distributed	Comments
Low-sodium mustard	Cellu, Featherweight	Health food stores and some supermarkets	
Low-calorie margarine	Fleischmann's, Mazola, Imperial, Parkay	Supermarkets	The calories are lower, because margarine is whipped with water to double the volume.
Imitation sour cream	Penn and Quil, Knudsen	Supermarkets	Contains approximately half the calories of regular sour cream.
Low-calorie Italian dressing	Kraft	Most supermarkets	
Low-calorie Russian dressing	Wishbone	Most supermarkets	
Hot sauce	Tabasco, McHenny Company	Supermarkets	Only a small amount is needed for flavoring, keeping sodium content low.
Milder soy sauce	Kikkoman	Most supermarkets and Oriental markets	Has one half sodium content of most soy sauce.
Worcestershire sauce	French's	Supermarkets	Has the lowest sodium content of any brand to our knowledge.
Gelatin, flavored	D-Zerta	Supermarkets	
Low-calorie apricot marmalade Low-calorie orange marmalade	Kraft S&W Nutradiet, Slenderella, Smuckers	Supermarkets Health food stores	Contain half to a third of the calories of regular marmalade. Refer to nutrient counter for specific calories.
VEGETABLES			
Low-sodium canned vegetables	Monarch, Iris, Cellu, S&W Nutradiet	Most supermarkets and health food stores	Contains no added salt.
Low-sodium tomato juice	Cellu, Featherweight	Health food stores and most supermarkets	

Product	Brand	Availability	Notes
Low-sodium tomato paste	Cellu, Featherweight	Health food stores and some supermarkets	
Tomatoes, whole	Cellu, Featherweight	Health food stores and some supermarkets	
EGG SUBSTITUTE			
Second Nature	Avoset Food Corporation	Supermarkets	Has only half the sodium content of most other egg substitutes.
FISH			
Dietetic canned fish, tuna, shrimp, salmon	Iris, Star-kist, Cellu, Chicken of the Sea, Van Camp	Most supermarkets	
NUTS			
Unsalted nuts	Planters	Most supermarkets	
Raw nuts		Health food stores	Have no salt or oil added.
Peanut butter, non-hydrogenated	Laura Scudder, Ralph's Old-Fashioned, Safeway's Old-Fashioned	Most supermarkets	
Peanut butter, unsalted	Peter Pan	Most supermarkets	
NON-DAIRY TOPPINGS			
Cool Whip	Bird's Eye	Supermarkets	Contain less calories and no animal fat.
Dream Whip		Supermarkets	
D'Zert Whip	Presto Foods	Supermarkets	Contains no artificial sweeteners. Only 8 calories per tablespoon.
Dieter's Gourmet Whipped Topping Mix	Dieter's Gourmet	Supermarkets	
STOCKS			
Beef	Cellu	Supermarkets and health food stores	Low in sodium content. For rich flavor we suggest you make your own. Refer to recipes in this book.
Chicken	Cellu	Supermarkets and health food stores	

Product	Brand Name	Where Distributed	Comments
STOCKS (continued)			
Frozen stocks	Jurgensen's	Jurgensen's, California	Low in salt content and has a rich flavor.
Vegetable	Cellu	Supermarkets and health food stores	
SUGAR SUBSTITUTE			
Granulated:			
Brown	Sugar Twin	Most supermarkets and some health food stores	Has a less bitter aftertaste than other brands in our opinion.
White	Sugar Twin	Most supermarkets and some health food stores	
Liquid	Sucaryl	Most supermarkets and some health food stores	We use Sucaryl when the preparation method requires heat. Saccharin is very heat sensitive; Sucaryl seems to be less so in our opinion.
Fructose		Health food stores	Refer to p. 295 for information on fructose.

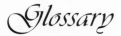

Calorie: A unit of heat measurement, or in terms of food, a measure of energy value of food.

Cholesterol: A fatlike waxy substance manufactured by the body and present in animal fats, oils, blood, bile, nerves, and all cells of the body. It is manufactured naturally by the body and also comes from foods we eat. The main dietary sources of cholesterol are foods of animal origin, such as liver, egg yolks, dairy products, most meats, shellfish, and some foods high in saturated fats. These lipids may undergo a chemical change and eventually may turn into fatty deposits. There is no cholesterol in foods of plant origin, such as vegetables, fruit, grains, and nuts. Buildup of cholesterol in the arteries has been associated with heart disease. Cholesterol is, however, important to the regulation of some body functions and as a precursor of vitamin D, sex hormones, adrenal hormones, and bile acids necessary for proper fat absorption.

Coronary Artery: Those arteries that supply blood to the heart muscles.

Coronary Artery Disease (Atherosclerosis): A condition caused by deposits, including cholesterol, which may decrease the inside diameter of the arteries and interfere with blood circulation.

Decalcification: Dissipation or loss of calcium from the bones, caused either by malabsorption of calcium or an inadequate supply of calcium in the diet, or binding of calcium by very large amounts of some fibers (phytates) in food, or inactivity.

Deficiency Disease: A disease resulting from an inadequate supply of nutrients needed by the body to function healthfully.

Diabetic Exchange: For diabetics who need to carefully calculate carbohydrates, fat, and protein intake to avoid sudden rises in blood sugar levels, the American Diabetes Association has devised a list of foods in which specific amounts are approximately equal in calories and nutrients as in the amounts of protein, carbohydrates, and fat. The list is divided into six main groups, or exchanges, for easy calculation: milk, vegetable, fruit, bread, meat, and fat.

Enriched: Foods to which nutrients have been added in amounts sufficient to restore those in the unprocessed state, as in bread enriched with iron, thiamin, and niacin to replace nutrients lost in the processing of the wheat.

Essential Fatty Acids: These are polyunsaturated and occur most abundantly in vegetable oils, such as corn oil. The body can neither manufacture them nor do without them. Fatty acids are essential for growth and certain body functions in infants and adults, as well. They also regulate serum cholesterol levels.

Fortified: Foods to which nutrients have been added in amounts sufficient to make the total content larger than that contained in the unprocessed state. Vitamin D, for example, is used to "fortify" milk.

Glucose: A single sugar occurring in fruit, honey and sugar, and metabolized by most cells of the body. Starch, a complex carbohydrate, breaks down to glucose.

Hemoglobin: A protein in the blood that contains iron and carries oxygen from the lungs to the tissues.

Hydrogenation: Combination of unsaturated fatty acids with hydrogen to form saturated fatty acids.

Hyper- (prefix): Excess.

Hypercholesterolemia: Abnormally high levels of blood cholesterol.

Hyperlipidemia: Abnormally high levels of blood triglyceride.

Hyperlipoproteinemia: Abnormally high levels of blood lipoprotein.

Hypertension: Abnormally high blood pressure.

Hypo-(prefix): Deficiency.

Insulin: A hormone made in the pancreas that lowers levels of blood glucose by stimulating its conversion into glycogen (starch). Insulin also promotes fat storage.

Lipid: A term used to cover all water-insoluble fats and fatlike substances, such as triglycerides, lipoproteins, steroids, cholesterol, and phospholipids.

Lipoproteins: There are two main types, both of which contain protein, cholesterol, and phospholipid. High density or alpha lipoproteins (HDL) contain a higher proportion of phospholipids and protein. Low density or beta lipoproteins (LDL) contain a higher proportion of cholesterol. Recently, too much LDLs have been associated with buildup of cholesterol that can cause heart attacks.

Malnutrition: An imbalance between the body's supply of nutrients and the body's demand for nutrients.

Metabolism: The chemical changes that go on in the body as food is converted into body tissue.

Nutrients: Individual chemical substances in foods that are used to nourish the body.

Plaque: A material deposited in arteries containing lipids, among other substances.

Polyunsaturated Fatty Acids: Generally, these are oils in their natural states and are of vegetable origin. Most vegetable oils are polyunsaturated, such as safflower, sunflower, corn, soybean, and cottonseed oils. The exceptions are coconut and palm oil.

RDA: The Recommended Dietary Allowances developed by the Food and Nutrition Board of the National Academy of Sciences during World War II is a table of nutrients in varying amounts for each age group considered as standards for optimal health.

Risk Factor: An inherent or environmental factor that is associated with increased incidences of coronary heart disease, but not necessarily the cause.

Saturated Fatty Acids: Saturated fats are usually of animal origin and solid at room temperature. Foods high in saturated fats include heavily marbled and fatty meat, whole milk and cream, cheese made from whole milk, and chocolate. The body also makes its own fat from excess food and this fat is predominantly saturated. Because coconut oil is a highly saturated vegetable fat, it also falls in the saturated fat category. Some foods, however, are higher in saturated fats than others.

Snack Foods: A loose definition of foods broadly considered to be of minimal nutritional value. These foods are generally high in sugar and/or fat content, such as potato chips, candy, and soft drinks.

Sodium: An essential mineral for life of man, animal, and plant. Sodium occurs naturally in many foods, but the principal source in man's diet is sodium chloride — ordinary table salt — of which sodium is one of the constituents. Sodium is important for many body functions, including temperature regulation. When excess sodium cannot be excreted by the body, it causes water retention, which puts a strain on various body organs. High sodium intake has also been associated with high blood pressure and the reduction of dietary sodium has been shown to reduce blood pressure.

Sucrose: Ordinary cane sugar. A disaccharide, sucrose consists of two molecules, one each of glucose and fructose.

Bibliography

American Medical Association, Phil L. White, Sc.D., ed. *Let's Talk About Food*. Publishing Science Group, Inc., 1977.

Church, Charles Frederick, and Church, Helen Nichols. *Food Values of Portions Commonly Used*. Philadelphia: J. B. Lippincott Company, 1975.

Goodhart, R., and Shils, M., eds. *Modern Nutrition in Health and Disease*. Philadelphia: Lea & Febiger, 1973.

Kraus, Barbara. *The Dictionary of Calories and Carbohydrates*. New York: Grosset & Dunlap, Inc., 1973.

Kraus, Barbara. *The Dictionary of Sodium, Fats, and Cholesterol*. New York: Grosset & Dunlap, Inc., 1974.

Lawler, Marilyn, and Robinson, Corinne H. *Normal and Therapeutic Nutrition*. New York: Macmillan Company, 1977.

National Dairy Council. *Guide to Good Eating*. Rosemont, Illinois. 1977; Nutrition Source Book, 1970.

United States Department of Agriculture. *Handbook of the Nutritional Contents of Foods*. New York: Dover Publications, Inc., 1975.

United States Department of Agriculture. *Composition of Foods*. Agricultural Handbook No. 8. United States Government Printing Office, 1963.

Recipe Index

A

Abalone Meunière, 83
Albondigas Soup, 27

APPETIZERS
  Appetizer Artichokes, 16
  Champagne Meatballs, 17
  Chicken Pacifica, 17
  Crab Dip, 13
  Guacamole, 14
  Marinated Mushrooms, 163
  Melon with Port, 18
  Pears Alexander, 225
  Pizza, 19
  Pizza Canapés, 20
  Scallops Dejonghe, 20
  Seafood Cocktail, 21
  Seafood Dip, 14
  Sirloin Teriyaki, 21
  Skinny Dip, 15
  Stuffed Cherry Tomatoes, 23
  Stuffed Mushrooms, 22
  Tortilla Salad, 24

APPLES
  Apple-Onion Stuffing, 99
  Applesauce, 199
  Apple Sizzle Crêpes, 231
  Apple-Stuffed Pork Chops, 118
  French Apple Tart, 218
  Waldorf Salad, 170

Apricot Ice Cream, 230
Artichokes, Appetizer, 16

ASPARAGUS
  Asparagus Picante, 138
  Steamed Asparagus, 138

Autumn Salad, 171

AVOCADO
  Avocado-Orange Salad, 167
  Avocado Salad, 157
  Guacamole, 14

B

Baklava, 213
Barbecued Chicken, 89
Basil Dressing, 177

BEANS
  Green Beans Amandine, 142
  Savory Green Beans, 147

Béchamel Sauce (White Sauce),
  187

BEEF
  Beef Brochette, 107
  Beef Stock, 39
  Beef Tacos, 107
  Champagne Meatballs, 17
  Chateaubriand, 108
  Chinese Beef with Pea Pods,
    109
  Roast Beef au Jus, 110
  Sirloin Teriyaki, 21
  Steak Diane, 111
  Steak Dijon, 112
  Steak Oscar, 112
  Tournedos Rossini, 113
  Vienna Dip, 110

BERRIES
  Berries on Ice, 228
  Berry Bowl, 222
  Chilled Berry Soup, 37

BEVERAGES
  Bloody Mary, 239
  Breakfast Shake, 239
  Eggnog, 240
  Herb Tea, 241
  Ice Ring, 242
  Mimosa Cocktail, 241
  Persian Refresher, 242
  Sparkling Punch, 242
  Sunrise Punch, 243
  Virgin Mary, 239
  Virgin Spritzer, 244

Wine Spritzer, 243
Yogurt Smoothie, 244

Biscuits, Cloud, 45
Blender Béarnaise, 188
Bloody Mary, 239
Blossom Peach Salad, 170
Bouquet Garni, 202

BREADS
  Bread Sticks, 49
  Cloud Biscuits, 45
  Corn Bread, 47
  Crescent Rolls, 46
  French Bread, 49
  Garlic Bread, 48
  Holiday Bread, 50
  Mexican Bread Pudding, 220
  Pizza, 19
  Pizza Canapés, 20
  Popovers, 51
  Ramona's Rolls, 53
  Ramona's Whole Wheat Bread, 52

Breakfast Shake, 239
Broccoli alla Romana, 139
Butter, Low-Calorie, 207
Buttermilk-Cucumber Dressing, 177

C

CABBAGE
  Coleslaw De Luxe, 160
  Gingham Salad, 163

California Cheesecake, 214
California Quiche, 62
California Salad, 167
California Tostada, 158
Candied Sweets (potatoes), 150
Cannelloni, Kathy's, 125
Cannelloni Noodles, 126
Cantaloupe Crab Boats, 168

CARROTS
  Carrot Cake, 219

Index   307

Index   309

310   Light Style

Sea Bass, Poached, 77

SEAFOOD
Abalone Meunière, 83
Cantaloupe Crab Boats, 168
Classic Sole, 75
Crab Dip, 13
Crab-Stuffed Sole, 82
Crêpes St. Jacques, 68
Dilly Trout in a Pouch, 76
Fish Stock, 41
Lime-Laced Lobster Tails, 84
Lobster Bisque, 33
Marine Kebabs, 77
Picnic Lobster, 85
Poached Sea Bass, 77
Scallops Dejonghe, 20
Scallops in Cider, 85
Scallops Marcus, 86
Seafood Cocktail, 21
Seafood Cocktail Sauce, 208
Seafood Dip, 14
Sole Amandine, 79
Sole Veronique, 81
Swordfish Piquant, 80
Whitefish à la Port, 82

Shredded Zucchini, 148
Sirloin Teriyaki, 21
Skinny Dip, 15
Snowdrop Cookies, 220

SOUFFLES
Chocolate, 233
Lemon, 234
Mushroom, 60
Spinach, 61
Strawberry, 235

SOUPS AND STOCKS
Albondigas Soup, 27
Beef Stock, 39
Chicken Soup Klara, 28
Chicken Stock, 40
Chilled Berry Soup, 37
Chilled Crookneck Soup, 38
Chinatown Soup, 29
Consommé Madrilène, 30
Court Bouillon, 78
Fish Stock, 41
French Onion Soup, 31
Gazpacho Andaluz, 39
Hearty Minestrone, 32
Lobster Bisque, 33
Pea Soup, 34
Potato & Leek Soup, 35
Turkey Stock, 40
Vegetable Soup, 36
Veal Stock, 39

Soy Sauce, 209
Spaghetti with Italian Meat Sauce, 129
Spanish Omelet, 59
Spanish Rice, 131
Spanish Sauce, 194
Sparkling Punch, 242
Spices and Herbs, 281-285

SPINACH
Creamed Spinach, 142
Crêpes Florentine, 67
Gingham Salad, 163
Lemon Spinach, 144
Spinach Soufflé, 61

STEAK
Steak Diane, 111
Steak Dijon, 112
Steak Oscar, 112
Tournedos Rossini, 113

Steamed Asparagus, 138
Steamed Rice, 132
Stocks. See Soups and Stocks

STRAWBERRIES
Strawberries in Meringue, 226
Strawberries Romanoff, 227
Strawberry Crêpes, 232
Strawberry Ice, 229
Strawberry Ice Cream, 231
Strawberry Sauce, 202
Strawberry Soufflé, 235

Stuffed Baked Potatoes, 153
Stuffed Cherry Tomatoes, 23
Stuffed Mushrooms, 22

STUFFINGS
Apple-Onion Stuffing, 99
Herb-Corn Bread Stuffing, 102

Suiza Sauce, 92
Sunshine Salad, 172
Swordfish Piquant, 80
Syrup, Rosewater, 214

T

TARRAGON
Chicken Tarragon, 97
Tarragon Sauce, 198

Tartar Sauce, 210

TOMATOES
Italian Tomato Sauce, 193
Stuffed Cherry Tomatoes, 23

Tomato-Cauliflower Salad, 165
Tomato-Mushroom Salad, 166
Tomato Purée, 195

Tortilla Salad, 24
Tournedos Rossini, 113
Trout, Dilly in a Pouch, 76

TURKEY
Roast Turkey with Royal Glaze, 99
Stock, 40
Turkey Crêpes Divan, 67
Turkey Divan, 98
Turkey Tetrazzini, 100

V

Vanilla Ice Cream, 230

VEAL
Veal Abel, 115
Veal alla Marsala. See Chicken
alla Marsala
Veal Bourguignonne, 116
Veal Parmigiana, 116
Veal Picatta. See Chicken Piccata
Veal Stock, 39
Venetian Veal, 117

VEGETABLES
Appetizer Artichokes, 16
Asparagus Picante, 138
Broccoli alla Romana, 139
Candied Sweets (potatoes), 150
Carrot Cake, 219
Carrots à l'Orange, 139
Cauliflower in Lemon Sauce, 140
Chantilly Potatoes, 151
Chilled Crookneck Soup, 38
Chinese Stir-Fry Vegetables, 141
Coleslaw De Luxe, 160
Creamed Spinach, 142
Crêpes Florentine, 67
Cucumbers in Yogurt, 160
Endive-Watercress Salad, 161
Fabulous Salad, 162
French Onion Soup, 31
Gingham Salad, 163
Green Beans Amandine, 142
Herbed Crookneck Squash, 143
Lemon Spinach, 144
Marinated Mushrooms, 163
Mediterranean Salad, 164
Minted Baby Carrots, 144
Mushroom Sauté, 145
Mushroom Soufflé, 60
Orange-Cauliflower Salad, 164
Oriental Omelet, 59
Oven-Fried Potatoes, 151